AIDS AND DRUG MISUSE

How important *is* the connection between the misuse of drugs and the spread of HIV infection? What impact has the arrival of AIDS had on the way we respond to health and social welfare problems?

HIV and AIDS have brought an unprecedented crisis to all those engaged in the provision of health and social services. Conventional wisdom and old methods have had to be re-examined critically; new problems have called for new information and new skills.

AIDS and Drug Misuse provides a major evaluation of the challenge of AIDS. An impressive array of contributors, all of whom have international reputations in their fields, presents the only synthesis of the wide variety of issues in this complex debate. The book charts the development of the epidemic, and looks in detail at the different strategies being implemented around the world to try and contain it. It also explores the changing role of the drug worker of tomorrow and assesses the implications for future prevention of the spread of HIV among drug injectors.

AIDS AND DRUG MISUSE

The challenge for policy and practice in the 1990s

Edited by
JOHN STRANG
and
GERRY V. STIMSON

ROUTLEDGE

LONDON AND NEW YORK

First published 1990
by Routledge
11 New Fetter Lane, London EC4P 4EE
29 West 35th Street, New York, NY 10001

Reprinted in 1992

Typeset by LaserScript Limited, Mitcham, Surrey
Printed and bound in Great Britain
Mackays of Chatham PLC, Chatham, Kent

British Library Cataloguing in Publication Data

Strang, John
AIDS and drug misuse.
1. Man. AIDS. Role of drug abuse.
I. Title II. Stimson, Gerald V. (Gerald Vivian), *1945–*
616,9'792071

Library of Congress Cataloging in Publication Data

AIDS and drug misuse / edited by John Strang and Gerry V. Stimson.
p. cm.
Includes bibliographical references.
1. AIDS (Disease)–Epidemiology. 2. Drug abuse–Complications and sequelae. I. Strang, John. II. Stimson, Gerry V. (Gerald Vivian)
[DNLM: 1. Acquired Immunodeficiency Syndrome-epidemiology. 2. Acquired Immunodeficiency Syndrome—etiology. 3. Substance Abuse–complications. WD 308 A287736]
RA644.A25A344 1990
614.5'993–dc20
DNLM/DLC
for Library of Congress
89–70182
CIP

ISBN 0-415-03099-4
0-415-05328-5 (pbk)

CONTENTS

ILLUSTRATIONS

FIGURES

TABLES

CONTRIBUTORS

Annette Barratt, Special Projects Officer, Phoenix House, London, England.

Ray Brettle, Consultant Physician, City Hospital, Edinburgh, Scotland.

Ernst Buning, Psychologist, Drug Department of the Municipal Public Health Service, Amsterdam, Netherlands.

Manuel Carballo, Chief, Social and Behavioural Research, Global Programme on AIDS, World Health Organization, Geneva, Switzerland.

Lesley Cooke, Development Director, Phoenix House, London, England.

Don C. Des Jarlais, Co-ordinator for AIDS Research, Narcotics and Drug Research Inc., New York, USA, and Director of Research for Chemical Dependency Institute at Beth Israel Medical Center and Guest Investigator at Rockefeller University.

Kate Dolan, Research Fellow, Centre for Research on Drugs and Health Behaviour, Charing Cross and Westminster Medical School, London, England.

Martin C. Donoghoe, Research Fellow, Centre for Research on Drugs and Health Behaviour, Charing Cross and Westminster Medical School, London, England.

Nicholas Dorn, Development Director, Institute for the Study of Drug Dependence (ISDD), London, England.

Richard Elion, Physician, Department of Social Medicine, Montefiore Medical Center, New York, USA.

Michael Farrell, Research Senior Registrar in Psychiatry, Addiction Research Unit, Institute of Psychiatry, London, England.

Samuel R. Friedman, Principal Investigator, Narcotic and Drug Research Inc., New York, USA.

Massimo Di Giannantonio, Psychiatrist and University Assistant, Drug Addiction and Alcoholism Unit, Institute of Psychiatry and Psychology, Universita Cattolica del S. Cuore, Rome, Italy.

Karen Gowler, Hospital Liaison Officer, Borough of Lambeth, London, England.

John Green, District Psychologist, St Mary's Hospital, London, England.

Timothy Harding, Chargé de Cours, the University Institute of Legal Medicine, Geneva, Switzerland.

David Hawkins, Consultant Physician, Genito-Urinary Medicine, Kobler Centre/John Hunter Clinic, St Stephens Hospital, London, England.

Rachel Lart, Research Worker, Monitoring Research Group, Goldsmiths' College, London.

Andrew R. Moss, Department of Epidemiology and International Health, San Francisco General Hospital, University of California, San Francisco, USA.

Bill Nelles, General Practitioner Training Officer, West Berkshire Health Authority, England. (Previously with the Terrence Higgins Trust.)

Robert Power, Senior Research Fellow, Centre for Research on Drugs and Health Behaviour, Charing Cross and Westminster Medical School, London, England.

Geof Rayner, Health Liaison Officer, Borough of Lambeth, London, England.

Giovanni Rezza, Consultant, Social and Behavioural Research, Global Programme on AIDS, World Health Organization, Geneva, Switzerland.

Massimo Riccio, Lecturer in Psychiatry, Charing Cross and Westminster Medical School, London, England.

Roy Robertson, General Practitioner, Edinburgh, Scotland.

Nigel South, Research Sociologist, Institute for the Study of Drug Dependence (ISDD), London, England.

Bruce Stepherson, Narcotic and Drug Research Inc., New York, USA.

Claire Sterk, Narcotic and Drug Research Inc., New York, USA.

Gerry V. Stimson, Director, The Centre for Research on Drugs and

Health Behaviour, Charing Cross and Westminster Medical School, London, England.

John Strang, Consultant Psychiatrist and Director, Drug Dependence Clinical Research and Treatment Unit, Bethlem Royal and Maudsley Hospital, London, England.

Meryl Sufian, Narcotic and Drug Research Inc., New York, USA.

Enrico Tempesta, Neuropsychiatrist and Associate Professor of Neuropsychopharmacology, Drug Addiction and Alcoholism Unit, Institute of Psychiatry and Psychology, Universita Cattolica del S. Cuore, Rome, Italy.

David Tomlinson, Executive Director, Phoenix House, London, England.

Jonathan Weber, Senior Lecturer and Honorary Consultant Physician, Royal Postgraduate Medical School, Hammersmith Hospital, London, England.

Alex Wodak, Director of Alcohol and Drug Service, St Vincent's Hospital, Sydney, Australia.

ACKNOWLEDGEMENTS

All contributors have agreed for their fees to be donated to PANOS, an international AIDS charity. We are deeply grateful to them for their generosity and for their tolerance as we have coaxed and cajoled them through tight schedules. We are especially grateful to Sheila Garnett, without whose patient secretarial support our editorial task would have been so much the greater. Finally, we owe thanks to all those who have helped us through our own personal reappraisal of attitudes and practices.

Part One

THE SIGNIFICANCE OF HIV AND AIDS

Chapter One

THE IMPACTS OF HIV: FORCING THE PROCESS OF CHANGE

JOHN STRANG AND GERRY V. STIMSON

The advent of HIV forces reappraisal: there is barely a field of science or care provision that will not be touched and will not be changed in the process. Just as the individual has to work through mixed reactions to the discovery of HIV status, so the scientific world, care providers and the general public must come to terms with the existence of the Human Immunodeficiency Virus and must also consider the various positive and negative impacts from the arrival of HIV. Not only is it incumbent upon us to undertake a fundamental re-examination of our attitudes and behaviour regarding this disease and drug use, but we must also conduct these without the luxury of adequate time. This re-examination must be conducted against the background of a ticking clock and the changing dynamics of the HIV epidemic.

Many still consider AIDS to be a disease that mainly affects gay men. Whilst this has been true – and continues to be true for many regions – we know from the experience of New York, Milan, Edinburgh and now Bangkok, that HIV infection can spread among drug injectors with alarming speed. Indeed, if current trends continue, injecting drug users will soon comprise the largest group of AIDS cases in Europe (World Health Organization 1989).

There is much about HIV infection and drug misuse that is shocking. However, our intention is not to shock, but to shock into re-examination. For those whose interests have been in the misuse of drugs, HIV has appeared as an unwelcome guest, in whose wake come hostility and prejudice from a general public who have only partially conquered their hostility and prejudice to drug-taking itself. Those whose interests have been in infectious and sexually transmitted diseases have been brought into contact with a new, marginalised clientele. Yet the response to HIV is bringing new perspectives, new scientific insights and new strategies for response, which themselves form the basis of this book.

We are at a point of change – a point of crisis between old ways of viewing drug problems and the new ones forced on us by HIV. The dimensions along which such changes are being considered provide the base from which this book emerges. In this rapidly growing field, heat often exceeds light as a characteristic of the debates: although this may be understandable, it does nothing to help bring about the necessary development of the paradigm that is now needed to understand and respond to drug use in the wake of HIV.

One feature of the crisis is the speed with which new information becomes available. At the present time this is outstripping our means of distribution of information and its assimilation. The whole sociology of knowledge is changing – not only are there new sources but there are also new types of information, much of which remains unpublished as yet or is out of date by the time it is published. There are now new journals being created specifically concerned with AIDS, and the development of electronic media for the rapid circulation of data. The investigation of AIDS is a truly international matter, and many researchers and practitioners now find their reference groups are international. In modern times, such a transition has never occurred with such rapidity. The knowledge required to understand and cope with AIDS has contradictory tensions – new scientific specialties emerge, old disciplines suddenly rise in status – and at the same time disciplinary boundaries must fade because no single discipline can comprehend the complexities. Behavioural scientists have to become knowledgeable about the work of virologists, immunologists and clinicians, and vice versa. Research methodologies once considered to be the esoterica of the social sciences suddenly become interesting to research funders seeking new ways to understand and respond to the epidemic.

Major re-examinations of policy and of services have been undertaken in many countries, such as the *Watkins Report* in the US (Presidential Commission on the Human Immunodeficiency Virus Epidemic 1988) and the reports (1988, 1989) from the Advisory Council on the Misuse of Drugs in the UK. Major changes of practice are also evident such as those seen in the Netherlands (see Chapter 14) and in Australia (see Chapter 12); and major projects – such as those co-ordinated by the World Health Organization (see Chapter 2) – are already in progress to map as well as steer these developments. This process of policy debate and learning is at an international level: new practices in Bangkok today might be picked up and adopted in Birmingham or Baltimore tomorrow. No one has simple answers or has solved the wide-ranging issues of prevention and care, but each has something to contribute by way of information, ideas or good practice.

AREAS OF CHANGE

Science

Whole new areas of science become relevant to the consideration of injecting drug use in the 1990s. These new areas include the study of blood-borne viruses and the development of drugs and vaccines which may prevent initial infection, may have an immunomodulating effect, or may be specifically antiviral in their activity. New insights are being gained into the virus and its replication; new tests and imaging techniques are being developed to permit study of HIV and other viruses, such as the polymerase chain reaction (PCR) test (see Chapter 3). There is also a much increased body of investigation into the relationship between viral replication, disease manifestation and psycho-biological influences.

Work is in progress on the development of tests which might act as markers of the disease status, some of which will be found to be predictive of HIV progression whilst others will merely reflect the duration of asymptomatic infection. Once effective antiviral treatments are developed and more routinely administered, then there will be a greater need for tests which indicate how advanced HIV disease has become in an individual and which monitor the effect of the anti-HIV treatment.

Basic scientific work is required on the interrelationship between drugs misuse and the clinical development of HIV disease. Use of opiates and of cannabis, for example, has long been known to result in moderate impairment of immunological responses to infection, even in the absence of infections themselves associated with the drug use. However, this has not previously been regarded as of major clinical significance and it remains to be seen whether – and if so, in what way – this alters the progression of HIV disease.

Medicine

Not only is HIV a new virus with its own particular characteristics which will themselves have an impact on the practice of medicine, but it is also associated with the appearance of hitherto rare clinical conditions such as Kaposi's sarcoma and systemic candidiasis, and even with new conditions, such as hairy cell leukoplakia (see Chapter 4). Both textbooks and practitioners will need to take on much new information over the next few years; and those that fail to do so will look sadly out of date.

New treatments are already appearing for the illnesses associated with HIV disease as well as treatments which specifically target the HIV virus itself, and we are beginning to learn of the important role played by co-factors in the progression of HIV disease. Herpes simplex, syphilis, cytomegalovirus and others have already been implicated, as have physical features such as genital ulceration and concurrent treatments such as steroid therapy – all have been identified as possible factors which increase the likelihood of infection or progression of HIV disease. Diseases which had previously been widespread but have in recent decades been reduced to the level of somewhat rare and eminently treatable conditions are now once again reappearing in the immunocompromised, HIV-infected individuals. Tuberculosis and syphilis, for example, are once again infections whose presence must be prominently considered and whose early and effective treatment is essential.

We (the editors) have adopted the term 'HIV disease' in preference to AIDS. As knowledge of the various manifestations of this disease increases, so it becomes clear that the clinical case definitions of AIDS (see Chapter 4) fail to describe the range of health problems that may occur to someone who has become infected with HIV. The *Watkins Report* (Presidential Commission on the Human Immunodeficiency Virus Epidemic 1988) in the US declared that the term 'AIDS' is obsolete. We prefer the generic term 'HIV disease' to cover the full range of HIV-related conditions from infection to AIDS.

It remains to be seen what factors will be relevant to the drug-using and former drug-using populations. Some features will undoubtedly be the same as those identified in homosexuals, but there are also likely to be differences because many people who inject drugs experience other infections from injecting with unsterile needles. What, for example, will be the effect on HIV disease progression of the wide extent of Hepatitis B infection amongst injectors, some of whom are chronic carriers with residual active Hepatitis B virus and some of whom will have superimposed delta virus?

Study of epidemics

Analysis of the HIV epidemic involves study not only of the time of arrival of the virus, but also its pattern and rates of spread and the extent of eventual penetration of different sections of the population. It now appears that some of the transmission amongst injecting drug users may reflect heterosexual transmission and not solely needle-sharing transmission as had previously been presumed. What are the behaviours and factors which influence the rate and extent of transmission, and might there also be protective factors? The fact that the virus has spread so rapidly in communities such as New York City (Chapter 8) and Edinburgh (Chapter 9) indicates that there is still much to learn about the interaction between HIV, populations and risk behaviours.

The combined study of HIV and drug misuse results in an interesting analysis of this part of the HIV epidemic, for there are complex relationships between the different behaviours. After all, it is not drug use *per se* which places the individual at risk of HIV infection – nor even injecting itself. Even sharing of equipment such as needles and syringes does not put the individual at risk unless the partner (or partners) who lends them has the virus in his or her blood – and even in these circumstances the individual will only be at risk if they are further down the chain of sharing and if no adequate equipment-cleaning precaution has been taken.

Specific aspects of drug use and behaviours associated with drug-seeking now assume a special significance (see Chapter 6). Until recently needle sharing did not attract much interest even amongst those interested in the drug field. Descriptive accounts of needle sharing existed in earlier times (e.g. Howard and Borger 1974) but they were not the subject of particular interest. Similarly, the association between drug use and sexual activities (and prostitution in particular) assumes a new importance – in particular, the possibility that drug use might be associated with a greater willingness to engage in high-risk sexual activity (such as unprotected vaginal or anal intercourse) has been mooted but has not yet been demonstrated. In addition, there are female drug users who may engage in more-than-usually-casual sex in exchange for drugs and who might be less likely to receive health education advice through prostitute networks.

Consider too the widespread concern about the rapid dissemination of new patterns of drug use and new drugs. The popularity of free-base cocaine and of crack in the USA and of inhaling heroin by 'chasing the dragon' in the UK are areas of legitimate major concern, although neither practice carries the risk of HIV infection through possible needle sharing. Yet in the longer term such behaviours could lead to a larger number of individuals who graduate to injecting their drug, or move into high-risk sexual behaviour such as prostitution to fund their drug use, hence placing themselves and/or others at increased risk by virtue of this previously unrelated drug use.

Travel also may have a significant influence on the pattern of the epidemic. The mobility of drug injectors within and between countries takes on a new importance. A migrant drug injector who does not have HIV may be at higher risk of infection by visiting areas where seroprevalence is high, and conversely a drug injector with HIV infection may import the virus to a new community. What is the frequency and duration of the travel? Over what distances? And with what degree of integration into the host drug-using community? Of particular practical significance is the extent to which malleable factors may contribute to this travel – for example, the move or regular inter-city travel of those addicted to heroin to adjacent cities or countries in which police attitudes or the availability of treatment may appear more attractive. Those with better services are likely to attract more people, but the cost of caring for the sick drug user may lead countries to reassess the extent to which they offer services to migrating drug users.

Education

A wide range of levels of risk behaviour exists across the community. Any proposal for an educational or public health information approach must consider the different impacts that might result at three distinct levels – on the general public, on the potentially at high risk, and on the actually at high risk. At the basic level, the general public rightly expect to be informed of changes in the dangers to which they are exposed, and of increases in our knowledge about these dangers. It is hoped that through the provision of knowledge there will be a shift in attitudes resulting in change in behaviour. At another level, this knowledge-attitude-behaviour change is particularly important to those already engaging in high-risk activities (in this context, certain injecting and sexual activities) and special information and educational programmes may target such individuals.

Between the general population and those who are already at high risk by virtue of their present behaviour, it might be useful to consider those individuals who could reasonably be regarded as at greater-than-average risk of moving on to high-risk behaviour, even though it is not presently within their repertoire. This latter group might cover individuals who are free-basing cocaine, smoking heroin, or sniffing amphetamine in large quantities and who might move on to injecting; those who are already engaging in atypical behaviour such as shoplifting to fund their runaway habits and who might move on to prostitution; and those who agree to participate in atypical sexual or drug-taking behaviour while in prison.

There must also be a reassessment of the targets for change. There are often powerful cultural, social and economic reasons why people engage in risk-laden behaviour. Helping drug users to change is not only about targeting individuals, but also about helping drug-using communities to change (see Chapter 16). It is clear that a behaviour change in the gay population occurred through existing mutual help systems which enabled the community to respond. Whether this dynamic will occur among injecting drug users is the key question. Whilst many projects target individual clients, some projects will also aim through them to enable wider changes in the community.

New terms in our vocabulary need clarification. For example, there has been much recent discussion about outreach work, but there are different ideas about what this entails. For some, the aim of outreach is to reach out and pull people into services; for others, the aim is to take expertise, resources and information out into the community.

Planning the response

To a large extent, the behaviour changes required for the benefit of individual health are also those that improve public health; but there is potentially a deep rift between considerations of personal freedom (and a right to exercise that freedom) and public calls to isolate those who are infected behind a cordon sanitaire, such as the one that was established in Cuba with the creation of the Los Cobos colony for all those found to be HIV positive in the compulsory national testing programme.

In planning responses, it is now clear that special attention must be paid to certain key behaviour changes – in particular, the cessation of sharing needles and syringes and the move from injecting to oral-only use, and the adoption of safer sexual practices. Existing services must be realigned and new services developed specifically in order to promote these changes. If greater change than this can be achieved, then so much the better, but the pursuit of higher-level goals must not be allowed to obscure the great benefits to both individual and public health that will result from the achievement of these intermediate goals (see Chapter 19).

Active recruitment is required. In the past, most drug services have adopted a passive approach to service delivery. The drug taker was expected to seek help; then, and only then, would consideration be given to providing help. With the arrival of HIV, a co-ordinated response must include strategies to contact and influence the broader drug-using constituency and not just those who specifically seek help. The prescription of drugs might be one way to attract people to drug treatment services, and there has been considerable debate about a new role for prescribing. But it is as well to remember that the prescription of drugs is not the only service which might attract the out-of-contact drug user. A recent study of help-seeking in London drug users (Drug Indicators Project 1989) found a wide range of services which out-of-contact drug users identified as potentially attractive – for example, general health care rated as highly as the provision of a prescription. In many countries – Sweden and Norway are good examples – a high proportion of the drug-using population is contacted by outreach workers without using methadone as a bait.

Planners might benefit from considering drug services as if they were a business. Although it is important to ensure that established customers continue to use the service as before, is there scope for capturing more customers from the out-of-contact population? Having drawn them into the sales room, is it possible to achieve sufficient retention that they are influenced by the product and use it? And do they then move on out of the premises, indicating that they are better for having received it and also leaving behind them vacant spaces for future customers? New approaches are currently being used in the broader range of drug services today, and there may be benefit in considering them according to their influence on these three functions.

In the new HIV-conscious drug services, attention must be paid particularly to the capacity of services to promote key changes in behaviour in the maximum possible number of people, while minimising the deleterious effect on other drug users. Today's planner is required to adopt an approach of therapeutic Benthamism.

Several of the chapters in this book describe new styles of work and new interpretations of the goals for work with drug users. In evaluating the potential worth of these approaches, it is important to remember that new and old approaches probably do harm as well as good. Therefore it is necessary for us to conduct a careful cost–benefit analysis of present and proposed action (and inaction), rather than just presuming that the interventions must necessarily be beneficial just because the staff are well intentioned. Some of the chapters in this book are speculative in nature and this is a reflection of the speed with which developments are taking place; it also illustrates the dilemma in which planners find themselves, for they are required to plan responses in the absence of performance indicators in the new projects.

Planning involves more than just providing for the drug user in specialist services. Effective prevention of HIV and the care of those with HIV disease entail a fundamental re-examination of the practices in a wide range of services: prevention and caring are also about provision of decent housing and support, and avoiding discrimination at the workplace and in the delivery of services (see Chapter 17).

Practical work with the drug taker

Major new areas of knowledge and practical skills are necessary in the new drug worker. It is not that the old knowledge and skills have been superseded; rather that there are now additional qualities which must be added to the requirements for the basic drug worker. No longer is it acceptable, in so far as it was ever acceptable, for drug workers to shrug their shoulders at descriptions of physical complications and suggest that the drug user should go to see a general practitioner. Drug workers must now regard physical deterioration or the results of blood tests as within their domain, and must also address uncomfortable subjects such as sexual behaviours and needle-sharing.

The profound changes required in the practice of the drug worker and the personal distress caused to staff by these changes should not be underestimated; they are perhaps only exceeded by the changes required in general hospital staff in adapting to dealing with drug users. Just as the drug taker may experience ambivalence when faced with the enormity of the changes required, and just as the drug taker may retreat into denial or rationalisation to avoid the work required in change, so these characteristics will be evident in the drug worker who is required to consider the rejected practice of yesteryear as part of the necessary practice of today.

Medical monitoring will undoubtedly be one of the important functions of the new drug worker. There is likely to be resistance to this notion as it may be seen as a return to a narrow medical model of understanding drug problems. Yet it would be a mistake to interpret the changes as a return to the old days, for that would fail to recognise that today's people, today's problems, and today's circumstances are different from those that existed yesteryear. When medical monitoring is considered as a key part of a holistic approach, then it becomes abundantly clear that the versatile drug worker should act as a medical watchdog. The drug worker will try to enhance drug users' own monitoring of their well-being, and conduct routine health checks, as well as keeping the drug user (as well as themselves) well informed on the significance of certain signs and symptoms (such as herpes simplex or candida infections) and the meaning of laboratory investigations. Once anti-HIV treatments become more widely used, then the drug worker is likely to be the most natural key worker fulfilling the co-ordinating role described in the second report on *AIDS and Drug Misuse* (Advisory Council on the Misuse of Drugs 1989), and this will necessitate a sound working knowledge of a much wider range of subjects, some of which are covered elsewhere in this book.

The importance of harm-minimisation interventions has rightly received much greater attention in the last couple of years. Many drug workers have undergone personal crises brought on by HIV in their clients, with the result that they have embraced harm-minimisation as an alternative to their previous abstinence-orientated work. However, full personal growth requires yet more change; the fully-fledged drug worker must be able to adapt his or her approach according to the circumstances and realistic potential for each individual drug user. Perhaps most challenging of all is the requirement to work at several levels simultaneously – for example, working towards abstinence or some other higher-level goal such as cessation of injecting while simultaneously exploring the protective strategies which the client would employ in the event of returning to more risk-laden behaviour. It may be that for many workers this challenge is too demanding; and organisationally it may be necessary to create different services in which staff are only required to work with a narrow repertoire of styles, rather than expecting each individual worker to be able to move competently across the entire range.

It is essential that appropriate attention is paid to the significant benefits that may be accrued from the achievement of intermediate goals. These may be particularly relevant for working with the drug user who is less clearly motivated to bring about any changes and who may easily be alienated by the identification of essential higher-level goals. Intermediate goals may not only be easier to achieve, but they may also be visibly more realistic so that the poorly motivated drug user is more likely to engage with the service. There is mounting evidence that many drug injectors are willing to adopt HIV-positive strategies and make changes that fall short of abstinence, but which could have a cumulative impact in levelling or reversing the epidemic curve.

CONCLUSION

No one will remain untouched by HIV over the next few years. HIV is forcing re-examination and change both for the individual and for society. We are at a point of crisis, but with destabilisation comes not only pain but also opportunity for change. Recognition of the constructive potential of crises long predates modern catastrophe or systems theories – indeed, the Chinese ideogram for crisis comprises two parts, one denoting danger and the other denoting opportunity. There is much about the arrival of HIV for which we should be grateful: the re-examination provides an opportunity for improvement in the quality and distribution of care across society and should result in alterations of attitudes and practices towards those who have so often been marginalised and have been poor consumers of health care. We are privileged that as a result of modern scientific study and communication we are well informed at a point in the HIV crisis when we have great opportunity to influence the unfolding course of the epidemic. Time will tell whether we have harnessed the creative force of crisis to its maximum effect. We can be sure that our successors will judge us harshly if we fail to respond constructively to this opportunity for change.

REFERENCES

Advisory Council on the Misuse of Drugs (1988) *AIDS and Drug Misuse Report: Part I*, London: Department of Health.

Advisory Council on the Misuse of Drugs (1989) *AIDS and Drug Misuse Report: Part II*, London: Department of Health.

Drug Indicators Project (1989) *Report on help-seeking and service utilisation*, London: Institute for the Study of Drug Dependence (ISDD).

Howard, J.A. and Borger, P. (1974) 'Needle sharing in the Haight: some social and psychological functions', in D. Smith and G.R. Gray (eds) *It's so good don't even try it once: heroin in perspective*, Englewood Cliffs, New Jersey: Spectrum Books (Prentice Hall).

Presidential Commission on the Human Immunodeficiency Virus Epidemic (1988) *Report*, Washington.
World Health Organization (1989) *AIDS Surveillance in Europe*, Quarterly Report no.20, Geneva: World Health Organization.

Chapter Two

AIDS, DRUG MISUSE AND THE GLOBAL CRISIS

MANUEL CARBALLO AND GIOVANNI REZZA

AIDS the epidemic was first recognised in the early part of the 1980s and is now affecting, to varying degrees but always in similar ways, every region of the world and virtually every country. AIDS the disease is in turn affecting some of the most fundamental aspects of human society, the ways in which it is organised, the way it functions and the manner in which it responds to health and social problems.

In the area of health and social planning one of the relatively immediate impacts of the global pandemic has been to highlight, more so than has been the case with any previous health problem, the complex cultural heterogeneity of contemporary society and the implications of that complexity for the development of health and social policies as well as the provision of services. Today, patterns of social organisation and the life-styles of cultural subgroups that have previously gone unnoticed or unremarked have, in the evolving context of AIDS, assumed a new significance. As much from the perspective of their role in defining the epidemiology of HIV transmission and AIDS as from the perspective of their life-styles and consequent needs, these characteristics have taken on a new degree of priority with regard to the formulation of public health strategies.

Nowhere has this been more evident than in the case of the transmission of HIV through sexual contact and drug injecting. In the case of the former, the AIDS epidemic has prompted a new mapping of the parameters of sexual behaviour and sexual preferences. Certainly, it has helped establish the social and political realities of homosexuality, its distribution within society, and the health and welfare needs related to it. More importantly, it has precipitated a societal recognition of the inherent strengths of, and opportunities within, a community whose members are coalesced around expressed values and self-help principles.

Approaches to the prevention and control of sexually transmitted HIV are still in the process of formulation and testing. The need to make condom use acceptable, feasible and, among particular groups, normative, will remain a challenge confronting health and social planners for some time to come. Improved knowledge about the sexual transmission of HIV, patterns of sexuality and the social and behavioural profiles of individuals and groups most at risk has nevertheless already demonstrated the importance of a planning process that is, at one and the same time, pragmatic and yet able to take into account the unique social characteristics of different groups.

The well-established association of HIV infection with drug-injecting behaviour now calls for an equally fundamental appraisal of the ways in which prevention and control policies and strategies can be designed to meet this aspect of the epidemic. For even if drug use has long been an integral part of many societies, and even if at different times in history it has prompted the development of control measures, never have the health and social implications of drug injecting been so far-reaching as in the context of HIV and AIDS, and rarely have they required such a profoundly new response as they do now.

NATURE OF THE PROBLEM

The need for new interventions to meet the problem of drug-injecting-related HIV and AIDS has confronted planners with the paucity of information currently available in this area and the fact that in many settings relatively little has traditionally been done to respond to the real health and social needs of drug injectors. The response of society to drug use has historically been one of rejection, disapproval and legal proscription: as a result, drug use has become a highly covert and poorly reported behaviour. Repressive laws, adverse publicity and the unsympathetic attitudes of the health sector as well as the public in general, have been met by a widespread reluctance on the part of drug injectors to participate actively and voluntarily in treatment programmes or to avail themselves of health and social services that might have provided support. Many of the same factors have probably contributed to a lack of creative action on the part of health and social services themselves and no doubt many opportunities for interventions have been missed or neglected. Given the nature of the AIDS pandemic and in the current climate of AIDS prevention and control, much of this needs to change.

Drug use in general has become more widespread than ever before and there is increasing evidence that the taking of drugs by injecting has become especially popular. In some communities injecting has become the primary route of drug use and, from a global perspective, the primary risk factor for HIV. In the United States, approximately 20 per cent of the more than 80,000 reported cases of AIDS are now directly associated with a history of drug injecting; if mixed cases where there is a combined history of both male homosexuality and drug injecting are included, the proportion rises to over 27 per cent. A similar overall distribution is emerging in Europe, where by 1989 approximately 27 per cent of all reported AIDS cases were related to a history of drug injecting but where in selected regions drug injecting accounted for as much as 50–60 per cent of all cases of AIDS.

Perhaps of even greater concern is the speed with which HIV infection can spread within communities where drug-injecting behaviour is common. In major cities such as Barcelona, Milan, New York and Edinburgh, the percentages of drug injectors known to have become HIV infected in the period of the epidemic range between 50 and 60 per cent (see Chapters 8, 9, and 10). In Rome and Amsterdam HIV seroprevalence rates associated with drug injecting have been reported to be in the order of 35 per cent (see Chapters 10 and 14), while in Belgrade, 44 per cent of the drug injectors who were tested as early as 1985–87 were found to have HIV antibodies.

Data from other regions, moreover, suggests that drug injecting is no longer a phenomenon of industrialised society alone and that it carries with it the same risk implications for HIV infection and AIDS. Although attention to the problem of drug injecting has traditionally focused on western countries, improved HIV and AIDS data from other regions has thrown new light on drug injecting. In Bangkok, Thailand, where only 32 out of the 3,180 drug injectors tested in 1987 were found to be HIV infected, the prevalence of infection among that same group was estimated to be over 40 per cent by early 1989. In Pakistan, India and Burma concern about HIV infection has provided new insights into the magnitude of the drug-injecting problem there too. In South America, 30 out of 188 serum samples obtained from drug injectors in São Paulo and Rio de Janeiro were confirmed to be seropositive; and in Argentina, 22 per cent of the 268 drug injectors examined between July and October 1987 tested positive.

The common factor in drug-injecting-related HIV infection increasingly appears to be the sharing of needles and syringes and, to a lesser extent, sharing of other drug-injecting equipment. As a critical factor in drug-injecting-related HIV transmission, needle and syringe sharing is both a primary and symptomatic problem: primary in the sense that this is where much of the initial exposure to the virus occurs and thus where many of the intervention strategies will need to be directed; and symptomatic to the extent that equipment sharing reflects other more fundamental and underlying problems.

Even in situations where the purchase of needles and syringes has long been possible through over-the-counter sales, drug injectors have often referred to their perceived unavailability and hence felt the need to loan or borrow equipment. Among the many factors that may have played a role, the social attitudes to drug injecting – especially among health workers, pharmacists, and others – may have, albeit unintentionally, made prevention and support services as well as needles and syringes, appear even more inaccessible than they actually were and thus may have contributed to the feeling of isolation and the need to share equipment. As 'gate keepers' these staff have traditionally been in a position to prevent or facilitate access to information, services and equipment. Opportunities for working constructively with drug injectors may have been poorly exploited as a result.

Legally and socially marginalised drug injectors have become distant from health and social services and have often been unaware of, or unwilling to use, the opportunities some services could have afforded, including counselling about personal and public health. Other factors, such as the relative cost of drug-injecting equipment, cannot be entirely discounted with regard to the decision to share needles and syringes. Nor can the fact that in many societies over-the-counter sales and other ways of providing clean equipment and reaching out to drug injectors have been traditionally hindered by a variety of legal, political and social constraints.

Placed in this broader social framework in which drug injecting has been stigmatised, actively prosecuted and associated with a range of other social problems, the sharing of needles and syringes may have gone on to represent, for some individuals, a symbol of group cohesiveness and solidarity and may have enhanced the process as well as the experience of drug injecting.

Drug injecting in the context of HIV infection and AIDS, however, has also become increasingly associated with a series of health as well as social problems. Diseases traditionally associated with drug injecting – for example, pneumonias, tuberculosis and endocarditis – appear to have become more widespread among drug injectors since the advent of AIDS. Moreover, what are now in fact cases of AIDS in which tuberculosis and pneumonia are opportunistic infections, may not be being diagnosed as HIV/AIDS related. Thus, currently reported AIDS cases among drug injectors may represent no more than a proportion of the true number of drug-injecting-associated cases (Stoneburner *et al.* 1988).

HIV infection among drug injectors also has other ramifications for society. In terms of secondary transmission, for example, even if the sexual partners of infected drug injectors are not themselves injecting, they are nevertheless at high risk of infection through sexual contact. Where there is already a high prevalence of HIV infection among drug injectors, the continuing risk of further transmission from this group to others represents a major problem. The potential for the sexual transmission of HIV to the non-drug-injecting community is heightened by the fact that prostitution is sometimes turned to by drug users as a means of financing drug purchases and also that many 'career' prostitutes are also occasional or regular injectors. In Amsterdam 83 per cent of 166 female drug injectors reported having been involved in sex for money (Van den Hoek *et al.* 1988). Similarly, prostitutes who inject drugs and share equipment are also exposed to HIV infection and their capacity to transmit HIV to their clients is a major cause of concern. Recent surveys of prostitutes diagnosed as having HIV antibodies were conducted in Florida, Seattle, New York and San Francisco. They found that 90 per cent of those interviewed had a history of drug injecting. The reduction of HIV transmission among drug injectors is thus important for the larger community as well as for drug users themselves.

Drug injectors also constitute a potential source of perinatal transmission. Over 50 per cent of all paediatric AIDS cases in the United States currently involve children of couples where one or both had a history of drug injecting (WHO Collaborating Centre on AIDS 1989); in Europe, of 509 children diagnosed as having AIDS 37 per cent were born to mothers with a known history of drug injecting (Centers for Disease Control 1989).

INTERVENTION STRATEGIES

Two critical needs have become apparent from this emerging global epidemiological picture. The first is the need to strengthen the primary prevention of drug-injecting behaviour and in so doing limit the numbers of people who might go on to be exposed to HIV infection. The second is to prevent secondary transmission of HIV. Unfortunately, primary prevention efforts have had only limited success to date. Programmes and activities involving drug legislation and law enforcement principles aimed at limiting the supply of illicit drugs have often been difficult to implement and sustain. In spite of the many efforts that have been made, the number of people injecting drugs for non-medicinal purposes is thought to be growing worldwide and currently stands at between 2,260,000 and 2,420,800 people. Despite their proven difficulties, however, interventions involving the prevention of drug supply have assumed high visibility and often priority importance in the eyes of both policy-makers and the public.

The second and perhaps equally important priority – namely, the need for action to prevent any further spread of HIV among drug injectors who, for whatever reason, are unable or unwilling to stop drug injecting – may well be where the real challenge in HIV prevention and control through the coming years will lie. Part of that challenge will be to define, test and implement strategies designed to reach individuals and groups who have previously gone unremarked and neglected, or whohave proved difficult to involve in risk-reduction or treatment programmes.

The difficulties involved in reaching drug injectors are well documented and new schemes now merit consideration. Some of these will need to build directly on the experience with previous initiatives such as methadone maintenance programmes while others will need to look to entirely new concepts of prevention such as making sterile needles and syringes more systematically available to drug injectors and reaching out with information, education and techniques for cleaning injecting equipment.

Some schemes are already being tried but on the whole are still in their infancy. The body of knowledge surrounding them still remains restricted to local health and welfare authorities, usually in cities with a known high prevalence of drug injecting. Many of them, moreover, have often been developed on an *ad hoc* basis in response to local crisis situations and as a result have not been explicitly designed or implemented with a systematic or in-built capacity for monitoring and evaluation. Their overall efficacy in preventing the further transmission of HIV is thus difficult to determine at this time, even though initial reports from the countries and local authorities in question suggest that the interim results are likely to be positive.

The attractiveness of these new interventions is due, in no small part, to their ability to respond to the diversity of needs presented by drug injectors. People with drug-injecting behaviour range from relatively young to old, involve men and women alike, and represent a variety of socio-economic, ethnic and cultural backgrounds. The fact that not all of them inject drugs regularly and that some do so on an intermittent and relatively unpredictable basis has often complicated already difficult prevention strategies. Schemes that seek to acknowledge this level of heterogeneity appear to be the ones that are having the greatest degree of acceptability. Thus, services that include the provision of food and shelter, occupational training, information, counselling and practical assistance in abstaining from high-risk behaviours, and provide medical and social care have generally been well received.

Among the more innovative schemes currently being tried are those that facilitate access to clean needles and syringes and other injecting equipment, and these are perhaps the most creative from a public health perspective. Their objective is specifically to reduce the need for and incidence of equipment sharing. Schemes that fall into this category have involved improved over-the-counter sales of needles and syringes at pharmacies and other paramedical facilities; the sale of needles and syringes through vending machines; the distribution of clean needles and syringes free-of-charge at designated sites, including mobile clinics; or needle and syringe exchange schemes.

Needle and syringe exchange programmes are especially attractive in that they involve the regular and routine collection of used equipment and thus radically reduce the risk of the sale or passing on of used materials. Programmes that have been based on a no-charge principle have been equally attractive to drug users, who are often short of money or are not especially motivated to purchasing equipment. The addition of counselling and the provision of advice and methods for family planning in conjunction with needle and syringe exchange appears to have enhanced the acceptability of these programmes. Outreaching beyond the confines of formal health or social welfare facilities has further helped professionals to make contact with drug injectors in a constructive and motivational fashion. All these activities have been further enhanced when anonymity and confidentiality have been ensured.

Although there is as yet no conclusive evidence that syringe- and needle-distribution schemes have had an impact on HIV infection rates, data from England, Scotland and the Netherlands suggest that these schemes are reaching drug injectors who have previously not been in touch with more conventional services (see Chapter 20). They have also proved useful in providing information, counselling and advice on drug use, sexual behaviour and HIV infection in addition to providing sterile equipment to individuals and groups who would not otherwise have sought such support.

Preliminary evidence from the Netherlands suggests that needle- and syringe-exchange programmes do not increase the rate of drug use or needle sharing, either among clients or among the wider community. Nor have they had an adverse effect on the demand for conventional drug treatment services. Indeed, they appear to have increased the demand by bringing larger numbers of users into frequent and positive contact with service providers.

Inevitably, one of the primary concerns and objections confronting new and innovative strategies such as those that facilitate access to clean needles and syringes is the moral and legal censure of practices that have traditionally been socially unacceptable.

Initiatives to provide needles and syringes, however, should not be seen in isolation and certainly not as exclusive. They are not meant to replace primary prevention initiatives but rather to reach those individuals who otherwise have not been motivated by primary prevention activities. As such, these approaches should be seen as complementary.

Methadone maintenance and other pharmacotherapeutic approaches may also be relevant. In the context of HIV infection and its association with drug injecting, the utility of methadone maintenance programmes and other pharmacotherapeutic schemes lies in the opportunity they provide for reducing the frequency of drug injecting, needle sharing and for providing a forum in which information, advice and counselling on safer drug use and sexual practices can be made available.

The effectiveness of these programmes, however, has been variable both within and between countries. As with other schemes, any overall assessment of their impact is difficult at this time but experience to date with methadone programmes in some areas – for example, New York City – suggests a relatively high dropout rate.

Methadone maintenance programmes have nevertheless often been successful in providing a basis for reaching drug users and providing information and counselling on HIV infection, safe sex and condom prophylaxis. In the Netherlands, up to 50 per cent of Amsterdam's 7,000 heroin addicts have been contacted annually through the city's methadone programmes.

There are, however, clinical and method-dependent limitations to the use of methadone. In the first instance, it is only appropriate in cases of opiate dependence and is not suitable for use in the case of other drug use. This in itself, given the increasing range of drugs being injected, is a major shortcoming. Moreover, while it can be useful in the treatment of regular opiate use it is not particularly appropriate in the treatment of intermittent drug use. Alone, it is insufficient in the management of opiate dependence and must be a part of a multi-faceted programme that includes education, counselling and other measures that support life-style changes, including abstinence.

CONCLUSION

Drug use in general, and drug injecting in particular, are now global problems. For a variety of health and social reasons they call for urgent and innovative attention. In the eight years that have elapsed since AIDS was first described, drug injecting has become a key factor in the epidemiology of HIV infection and AIDS. Needle sharing has emerged as one of the ways in which infected blood can be transmitted from one user to another. In communities where drug injecting is common, AIDS prevention and control programmes need to address this aspect of the problem.

Previous approaches to primary prevention have had only limited success and in recent years drug injecting has become more widespread than ever. The prevention and control of HIV infection, because of the broad health and social implications AIDS represents, may in many communities have to take precedence over the primary prevention of drug injecting. They should never be seen as mutually exclusive aims or strategies, however, for over the long term each has much to gain from the success of the other.

The complexities of drug injecting where needle sharing is a common feature of the behaviour, will not be easily overcome unless approaches to the problem are sensitive and respond to the needs of people who, for whatever reason, have not been able to – or do not want to – stop drug injecting. Secondary prevention or the prevention of HIV infection among drug injectors, if it is to be successful, will not only have to resort to new and creative methods but will also have to draw upon the support of broader political and social structures than are represented within the health sector alone. Their experience, skills and legitimacy will need to be brought together to take up this new global challenge.

REFERENCES

Centers for Disease Control (CDC Atlanta) (1989) Update: Acquired Immunodeficiency Syndrome – United States 1981–1988. *MMWR* 38: 229–36.

Stoneburner, R.L., Des Jarlais, D., Benezra, D. *et al.* (1988) 'A larger spectrum of severe HIV-1-related disease in intravenous drug users in New York City', *Science* 242: 916–19.

Van den Hoek, J.A.R., Coutinho, R.A., van Haastrecht, H.J.A. *et al.* (1988) 'Prevalence and risk factors of HIV infections among drug users and drug-using prostitutes in Amsterdam', *AIDS* 2: 55–60.

WHO Collaborating Centre on AIDS, Paris (1989) 'AIDS Surveillance in Europe', *Quarterly Report* No. 21, 31 March.

Part Two

UNDERSTANDING THE VIRUS AND DISEASE

Chapter Three

HIV: THE VIRUS AND LABORATORY TESTS

JONATHAN WEBER

THE DISCOVERY OF THE HUMAN IMMUNODEFICIENCY VIRUS

When AIDS was first identified as a new syndrome in 1981, various theories were put forward as to the possible cause. As it became clear in 1982 that blood transfusion could transmit AIDS, the theories that AIDS may be related to a specific homosexual problem – such as over-exposure to semen or recreational drugs – became untenable. Only an infectious agent could explain the observed transmission by sexual intercourse and blood inoculation; furthermore, the occurrence of AIDS in haemophiliacs who had been exposed only to plasma-derived clotting factors confirmed suspicion that only a virus could be responsible.

The search for the virus causing AIDS gathered momentum during 1983. A number of groups were convinced that AIDS might be caused by a retrovirus. Robert Gallo in Washington had been investigating animal retroviruses for 20 years; these viruses are widespread in the animal world, and cause a number of tumours and neurological diseases in animals as diverse as chickens and sheep. One particular retrovirus of cats, the Feline Leukaemia Virus (FeLV) causes not only leukaemia, but also an immunodeficiency unrelated to tumour development. This gave a potential clue to a retroviral cause of AIDS. Gallo had been searching for a human retrovirus as a cause of leukaemia for many years, without success. However, in 1980, his group isolated a novel human retrovirus from a rare T-cell leukaemia, which was named the Human T-cell Leukaemia Virus Type 1 (HTLV-1). The techniques derived to isolate this virus were then applied to AIDS.

Simultaneously, Luc Montagnier in France was attempting to isolate a retrovirus from the lymphocytes of an AIDS patient, and obtained a positive result in late 1982. Finally, in May 1984, Gallo and Montagnier succeeded in growing enough virus to make reagents which identified this virus, now called the Human Immunodeficiency Virus Type 1 (HIV-1), as the cause of AIDS and associated clinical conditions. (Old publications may refer to the virus as LAV-1 or HTLV-III – now called HIV-1.)

How does a retrovirus replicate?

A retrovirus is an RNA-containing virus which replicates through making a DNA copy of its genome. Retroviruses are classified into three groups: the oncogenic retroviruses, which cause cancers; the foamy viruses, which are widespread and even infect humans, but which are without any known disease association; and the lentiviruses, which include HIV. These lentiviruses (or 'slow' viruses) are so named because of their ability to cause disease some years after infection.

The HIV viral particle consists of an outer coat (the envelope), and an inner core structure. Within the core is the RNA, which contains the eight viral genes which encode the viral proteins of the envelope and core, and all of the viral enzymes which allow replication to occur. The proviral DNA copy is made by the action of viral enzymes – in particular, the reverse transcriptase enzyme. The DNA stage (the provirus) then integrates into the host cell chromosomes randomly, and will persist in the host's DNA for the life of the cell. Thus, these retroviral infections are persistent for the life of the host. The virus may go through long periods when it is apparently 'latent'. During these times, although the viral DNA has been integrated, it is not being transcribed into producing viral proteins. Certain factors, as yet undefined, can activate the viral replication, and the virus will enter a period of rapid replication which will lead to cell death, and a clinical effect. It is misleading to think of HIV as a 'latent' infection. At any one time, only a proportion of the virally-infected cells will be replicating HIV, and so the remainder of non-replicating cells will contain 'latent' virus. However, the virus is not latent in the body as a whole, as continuous low levels of HIV replication occur throughout infection. It is believed from cell culture experiments that concurrent or intercurrent infection with other viruses like cytomegalovirus (CMV) or herpes simplex, or the new HHV6, may activate HIV, and promote HIV replication, but this has not yet been identified in living subjects.

HIV infects cells in the body by the binding of the outer envelope of the virus to a particular molecule on the cell surface, called the CD4 antigen. Cells bearing the CD4 molecule are principally those of the immune system, particularly a subset of lymphocytes in the blood known as T-cells. Other immune-active cells (such as macrophages) and antibody-producing cells (B-cells) can also be infected by HIV. Cells which do not have the CD4 molecule on their surface cannot generally be infected by HIV. Although this model explains the infection by HIV once the virus is in the bloodstream, it is not easy to explain sexual transmission of HIV in virological terms. The virus must cross the vagina, to encounter CD4-positive cells, but whether the virus can cross intact skin is uncertain. While some animal evidence suggests that the virus can cross the vaginal walls, other studies in humans suggest that ulceration or abrasions of the genitals caused by sexually transmitted infections may enhance the spread of HIV. The virus binds to the CD4 molecule, and is then internalised into the cytoplasm of the cell. The viral reverse transcriptase then generates the proviral DNA copy, which enters the nucleus and integrates into the host DNA. New viral particles are produced by the action of the host's own DNA enzymes, which read off the viral DNA code to produce viral proteins. These proteins accumulate under the cell surface, and will bud off from the cell as mature, infectious virions which can go and infect new cells. If viral replication occurs at a controlled rate, the cell will survive, and chronically produce new viral particles. If there is unchecked replication, many new virions will be produced, but the cell will be killed; this is known as virally-induced cell lysis.

HIV infection of CD4-positive T-cells may therefore lead to lysis of these particular cells only. This virology fits in well with the clinical findings in AIDS patients, where it has been observed since the first cases that there is a specific reduction in CD4-positive T-cells in the blood. These CD4-positive T-cells are central to the functioning of the immune system. The death of these cells after many years of HIV infection leads to immune deficiency, and the appearance of the opportunist infections and tumours which is the clinical characteristic of AIDS.

What does a retrovirus look like?

The HIV virion (viral particle) is a spherical structure, just 120 nanometres (10^{-9}m) in diameter. The outer coat, the envelope, is formed from the cell surface of the infected cell from which the virus has budded, and is a lipid bilayer. Through this coat, virus proteins are expressed, and these envelope proteins are important as they are the only part of the virus available on the surface. It is the major envelope protein – known as gp120 – which binds to the CD4 molecule. The core of the virus consists of a geometric array of the p24 protein (the numbers refer to the molecular weight of the protein), and at least ten other minor proteins are produced in the mature virion. All of these proteins will be produced during infection by HIV, and all are antigens which can be seen by the host's immune system. Antibodies are therefore found to the principal antigenic proteins – gp120 and p24 – but also to the other minor proteins (see Figure 3.1).

Antibodies to these proteins appear within 6–12 weeks after infection, and generally persist for the life of the infected subject. The presence of HIV is currently measured by detecting the antibody response to the proteins of the virus – the 'AIDS test'.

The appearance of HIV-2

In 1985, a group of American researchers noticed that a population in Dakar, Senegal, in West Africa, were infected by a retrovirus which did not appear to be HIV-1. The antibodies found in these subjects partially reacted with HIV-1 proteins, but reacted more strongly with a lentivirus isolated from the lymphocytes of an Old World primate – the Simian Immunodeficiency Virus (SIV). Subsequently, this virus was isolated by scientists in France, and has now been termed HIV-2. This virus also causes AIDS, and is also restricted to infecting only cells expressing the CD4 molecule; however, it is possible that the interval of latency between infection and disease is longer. HIV-2 is still largely restricted to West Africa – in particular, Senegal, Guinea-Bissau, Ivory Coast, Gambia, Mali and Mauritania – and the Cape Verde islands. However, the virus is transmitted in the same manner as HIV-1 – by unprotected sexual intercourse and by blood transfusion (and hence presumably by sharing of contaminated injecting equipment by drug users) – and is thus spreading around the world. Cases of HIV-2-associated AIDS have been reported in many European countries, from subjects exposed to HIV-2 in West Africa.

Figure 3.1 The structure of the Human Immunodeficiency Virus

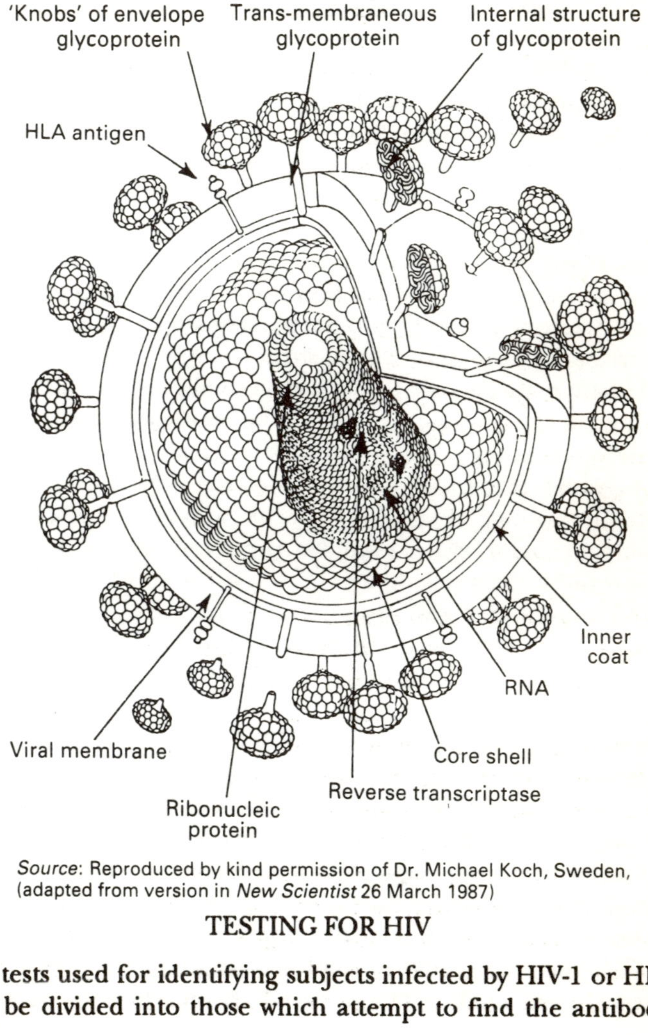

Source: Reproduced by kind permission of Dr. Michael Koch, Sweden, (adapted from version in *New Scientist* 26 March 1987)

TESTING FOR HIV

The tests used for identifying subjects infected by HIV-1 or HIV-2 may be divided into those which attempt to find the antibodies made against the viral proteins, and those which attempt to find the virus itself. The former are relatively simple tests, which can be used worldwide with increasing sensitivity (ability to find a positive result) and specificity (reactive only with genuine HIV infection). The latter tests on virus identification are considerably more specialised, and so less reliable at present.

Testing for antibodies

Screening assays

The great majority of subjects who have been informed that they are HIV positive have been found to have a positive antibody assay. Because HIV almost invariably causes an antibody response, antibody tests are reliable though indirect assays for the virus. The assays consist of a plastic well in which HIV is coated on to the surface of the plastic. Blood is taken from the subject, and allowed to clot in a tube. The clear fraction – the serum – is removed, and a small quantity is added on to the well coated with the HIV. After a short period, the serum is washed off. Any antibodies in the serum which are specific for HIV will remain bound to the virus, which is attached to the plastic. These antibodies are then detected by adding another antibody which reacts with all human antibodies, which is coupled to a marker (often a chemical which will result in a colour change). If specific anti-HIV antibodies are present, a colour change will be produced, which is called a positive result. This type of assay is known as an ELISA (Enzyme-Linked Immuno Sorbent Assay).

There are a number of different formulations of these assays, although all have broadly similar structures. The solid phase (the plastic well, described above) may instead be a plastic bead, or latex particles, and a number of different methods of antibody detection are available. Some more recent assays can be performed with just a drop of blood without the need to separate the serum, and others can be read in minutes. There is even interest in measuring these antibodies outside of the blood – for example, in saliva, where they occur at a lower concentration than in serum, but where it is more convenient to collect them. All require to be performed in a laboratory at present. However, all of these tests have a failing: any serum which binds to the plate will be recorded as positive. The problem is that some subjects, although perfectly well and not infected by HIV, may have odd antibodies in their serum which will give a positive reaction in these assays, when they should be negative. To avoid the possibility of false positives, most laboratories will test reactive sera with more than one type of assay; some sera will still be difficult to interpret and this requires confirmatory assays, in more specialised laboratories.

Confirmatory assays

The above screening assays are rapid, cheap and really quite reliable; they may have a specificity and sensitivity of over 99.5 per cent. However, if enough sera are screened, false positives (i.e. should really be negative, but come up positive in the screening assays) and false negatives (i.e. should be positive, but do not react) will be a problem. The greater problem is with the false positive sera; these require further tests, usually performed in a specialised central reference laboratory. Confirmatory tests use differing methods, in which the test serum has to compete with a standard serum, or other techniques. Some laboratories use a test known as the Western blot; this involves having the HIV viral proteins spread out on a nitrocellulose strip, where they are layered according to their molecular weight. The test serum reacts with these proteins, and when the strip is developed, specific bands appear which can be correlated exactly with reactivity with HIV. Any false positive will have a different pattern.

Testing for the virus

Examining the cells

It may take at least six weeks, and occasionally much longer, for antibodies to the virus to develop, and during this 'window' period, antibody-based tests may be negative. It is possible that some of these cases may be resolved by looking for an antibody to one particular HIV protein which appears first (the nef protein), but this remains a research manoeuvre. Most attempts to find HIV when antibodies are absent will depend on culturing the virus from the blood, or detecting the viral DNA genome by molecular biological techniques.

It seems that only one in every 10,000 lymphocytes in the blood is infected by HIV, which makes looking for the virus like looking for a needle in a haystack. Culturing the lymphocytes in a cell culture flask will allow the virus to multiply, until it is in sufficient quantity to be identified. This is a time-consuming assay, requiring considerable expertise, and is expensive to perform; in addition, there is only a 50 per cent chance of success in obtaining a positive culture.

Recent advances in molecular biology have finally made it possible to look for the HIV genome directly. By using a technique known as the polymerase chain reaction (PCR) it is possible to amplify by one million times a specific sequence of DNA. By multiplying the HIV DNA – even if it was present in small quantities initially – it is then possible to identify the DNA as being from HIV. This is a technique for identifying HIV directly, and should have exquisite sensitivity and specificity. However, as yet this is still a research technique, and there are teething problems with the fine sensitivity. Thus, it is not yet possible to rely absolutely on a PCR result, but the future for this technique is extremely promising and rapid progress is taking place in the refinement of this test.

Examining the serum

In addition to detecting the HIV genome, and antibodies to its proteins, assays have been developed to detect viral proteins themselves in the serum. The principal core protein – p24 – seems to be the easiest protein (or antigen) to find, and commercial tests are available. Most subjects who have detectable p24 antigen are those in the later stages of HIV infection; the finding of a positive p24 protein in the blood of asymptomatic subjects is associated with a higher probability of AIDS developing. However, only 70 per cent of patients with AIDS have detectable p24 antigen in the blood, and so this assay is not absolute. Levels of p24 will fall after successful therapy with zidovudine (AZT) and so this is a useful indicator of response to therapy.

PROGNOSTIC ASSAYS: MONITORING AND PREDICTING THE COURSE OF HIV-DISEASE

A number of different tests have been put forward as being of value in predicting which asymptomatic subjects will go on to develop AIDS most rapidly. The first indicator was the measurement of the number of CD4-positive T-cells in the blood; these are counted by staining with a specific antibody. CD4-positive cells decline gradually over time in HIV infection, and a fall to below 400 million/ml of blood is associated with a greater risk of AIDS developing. At levels of 200 or less, the subject is at high risk of developing opportunistic infections such as pneumocystis carinii pneumonia (PCP) (see Chapter 4). It is essential to perform serial assays so that the trend is observed, rather than rely too much on one reading.

The importance of serial readings applies to the other measurements which correlate to varying extents with prognosis. Antibodies to the core protein, p24, decline before AIDS develops, whereas antibodies to the envelope are maintained over time, and this discrepancy has also proved useful in predicting progression. Other measurements, such as elevation of beta-2 microglobulin or neopterin (products of damaged lymphocytes), have also been correlated with prognosis but their clinical value is not yet established (Moss 1988). At present, the most reliable indicators of the likely clinical course of HIV disease appear to be p24 antigen appearance, loss of anti-p24 antibody, elevation of beta-2 microglobulin – but most predictive of all, the loss of CD4-positive T-cells.

HIV was characterised only four years ago, and the commercial auxiliary assays are less than three years old. We are already developing 'third generation' ELISA assays that use more sensitive techniques and more specific reagents. The next five years will see complex research techniques applied simply in laboratories all over the world, so that HIV testing will become even more straightforward and reliable. However, it is also even more clear that we have not yet fully understood the complexity or the diversity of these viruses, and new developments will continue to reveal our ignorance until the next century.

REFERENCE

Moss, A. (1988) 'Predicting who will progress to AIDS', *British Medical Journal* 297: 1067–8.

Chapter Four

CLINICAL FEATURES OF HIV INFECTION AND AIDS IN DRUG TAKERS

RAY BRETTLE, MICHAEL FARRELL AND JOHN STRANG

The impact of HIV infection on drug services is slowly dawning. Drug takers have so far had poor access to and made poor use of both general health care facilities and drug treatment facilities. They are widely regarded as a poorly compliant group of patients who fail their appointments and default from treatment. The advent of HIV has set a new challenge to adopt a more flexible approach. Part of this flexibility requires good liaison between the different care providers in primary care, HIV clinics and drug services. However, an effective service response also requires all drug services to take on a more direct role in the physical aspects of patient care that have hitherto been neglected.

With time, the number of drug takers who are positive for HIV will increase, as will the number with symptomatic HIV disease. Individuals and families who so far have had to cope with drug problems and socio-economic deprivation are now being devastated by HIV infection. Despite the fact that drug users may form up to a quarter of the HIV-positive population there is little literature on their particular clinical problems.

The high morbidity associated with intravenous drug use is well recognised: subcutaneous abscesses, cellulitis, septicaemia, endocarditis and hepatitis are among the most common side-effects. Complications may be technique-specific or substance-specific. All of the above complications are technique-specific in that they are a direct result of the injecting practice itself. Additionally, substance-specific complications may occur: liver damage with barbiturates, psychosis with amphetamines or cocaine, and heart attacks after intravenous cocaine use. The infective nature of these widespread injecting complications are particularly significant in an increasingly immuno-compromised individual. For example, in Northern Europe in the 1980s, there were several outbreaks of systemic candida infection and candidal endophthalmitis (sometimes resulting in blindness), probably associated with use of old and contaminated lemon juice in the preparation of injectible blackmarket heroin (Hay 1986). Tuberculosis is now four times as frequent in New York heroin addicts who do *not* have AIDS, compared with four years ago. It might even be that attention to these complications may itself help to reduce the frequency of injecting drug use in this subpopulation.

The clinical features of HIV infection are now superimposed on those long-recognised physical complications. Despite the major differences in the broader management problems of the drug taker, many of the features of HIV monitoring and treatment of the drug taker are the same as in other risk groups.

THE DEFINITION OF AIDS

AIDS is not a single disease. The original description of AIDS was devised by the United States Public Health Centers for Disease Control (CDC) in Atlanta to provide a consistent definition to ensure uniformity of reporting. The definition of AIDS was adopted before the discovery of the aetiological agent, the Human Immunodeficiency Virus (HIV), and was based on the discovery of one or more opportunistic infections (described later) or conditions that were moderately indicative of cellular immunodeficiency in the absence of any other underlying cause. Although AIDS is the most commonly known outcome of HIV infection, people infected with HIV have a spectrum of clinical manifestations.

Many clinicians now find it more relevant to refer to HIV disease rather than AIDS, although classic AIDS remains important for uniformity of international reporting. A later CDC classification identifies stages of HIV disease progression (it is a hierarchical classification: see Table 4.1). After an initial acute viral illness (Group I), individuals may be completely asymptomatic with good immune function (Group II). They may then develop enlarged lymph nodes (greater than 1cm) in two or more non-adjacent sites (Group III). When there has been a significant decline in their CD4 count (below 400) symptoms usually become more serious, although some individuals may remain relatively well. AIDS Related Complex (ARC) is a term commonly used to describe a constellation of symptoms: it is now classified as Group IVa disease. This staging system is now used in clinical assessment, in research, and in monitoring the response to treatment. Classic AIDS falls into CDC IVc. As can be seen from Table 4.1, it is only part of the spectrum of HIV disease.

Table 4.1 CDC classification system for HIV

Group I:	Acute infection
Group II:	Asymptomatic infection
Group III:	Persistent generalised lymphadenopathy
Group IV:	Other disease
Subgroup a:	Constitutional disease
Subgroup b:	Neurological disease
Subgroup c:	Secondary infectious diseases
Category c1:	Unspecified secondary infectious diseases listed in CDC surveillance definition for AIDS
Category c2:	Other specified secondary infectious diseases
Subgroup d:	Secondary cancers
Subgroup e:	Other conditions

Source: CDC (Centers for Disease Control) 1988

Individuals with advancing HIV disease may also complain of vague constitutional symptoms or more general problems such as unexplained diarrhoea, fever (greater than 38 degrees centigrade) lasting longer than one month or unexplained weight loss of greater than 10 per cent of body weight. Some may complain of muscle or peripheral nerve problems or spinal cord problems. Central Nervous System involvement can be seen with acute confusional states or chronic impairment of intellectual functioning leading to dementia (see Chapter 5). Patients at this stage are prone to infections with organisms which do not usually cause serious illness in the absence of immunosuppression. Patients may also develop serious cancers specifically associated with HIV infection such as the skin tumour Kaposi's sarcoma and cancer of the lymph nodes (or glands) such as non-Hodgkins lymphoma or primary lymphoma of the brain. Kaposi's sarcoma occurs almost exclusively in homosexual HIV-positive patients.

From acute infection through to later stages of HIV disease

The full natural history of infection with HIV is still unknown. There are three primary routes of infection: sexual contact with an infected person; exposure to infected blood or blood products; or perinatally from an infected mother to her child (vertical transmission). Symptoms of the acute infection may appear two to six weeks after exposure to the virus and antibodies to HIV develop within three months (see Figure 4.1). These antibodies probably persist for life. The proportion of HIV-positive individuals who progress to symptomatic illness increases with time but the actual clinical course is very varied. In one cohort of seropositive drug takers followed for two years 12 per cent developed AIDS but their duration of infection was not known. The average incubation time (the time from original HIV infection to the onset of AIDS) is very variable but is usually in the order of eight to 12 years.

Clinical predictors of disease progression are still unclear. However, systemic symptoms such as fever, night sweats, weight loss, oral candida (thrush), hairy leukoplakia and herpes virus infection are associated with an increased likelihood of developing AIDS. Serial measurements of CD4-positive T-cells showing a fall below 400 or less are associated with a greater risk of AIDS developing (see Chapter 3). Other indicators are the appearance of the p24 antigen, loss of the p24 antibody and elevation of beta-2 microglobulin; however, some of these tests may primarily reflect the duration of infection.

The factors which influence the likelihood of initial infection or the rate of progression of HIV infection have not yet been confidently identified; various infections such as with the herpes simplex virus or CMV may act as co-factors by stimulating HIV replication (for a review, see Lifson *et al.* 1988). The influence of drug use on disease progression remains yet to be fully elucidated. Female drug injectors may be more likely to become HIV positive than their male counterparts; one New York study (Des Jarlais *et al.* 1987) found 58 per cent of female injectors to be HIV positive compared with 40 per cent of male injectors – although the reasons are still not clear. Recent work has suggested that there may be a genetic factor influencing the rate of disease progression (Lifson *et al.* 1988). It now seems that without treatment most people infected with HIV will become ill eventually.

Figure 4.1 Schematic representation of possible course of untreated HIV disease in a drug user

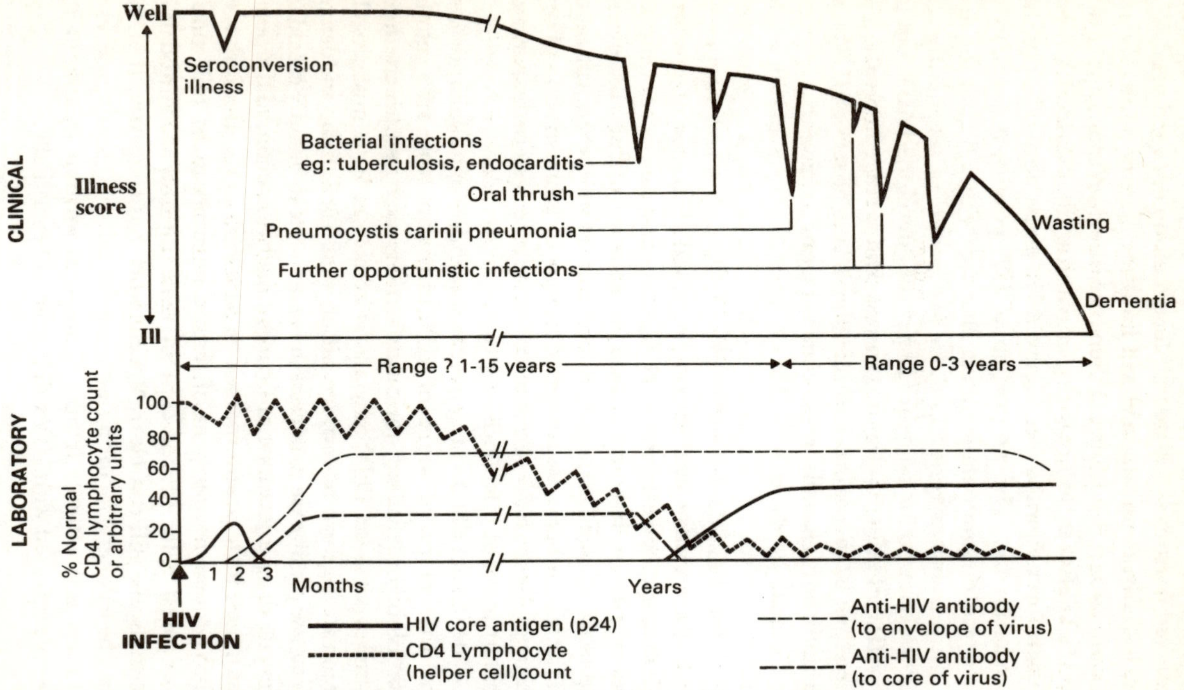

Source: Adapted, with permission, from an original by the Advisory Council on the Misuse of Drugs, 1988

OVERLAP OF DRUG AND HIV SYMPTOMATOLOGY: CLINICAL FEATURES BY SYSTEM

Assessment of the significance of certain symptoms often associated with HIV illness is complicated in the drug taker. For example, the opiate addict will frequently have night sweats and diarrhoea associated with the emergence of withdrawal symptoms, and is also likely to have lost weight due to drug-induced loss of appetite as well as poor diet (see Table 4.2).

Respiratory system

In AIDS the lung is the organ most commonly involved. Involvement can be due to infection, opportunistic or non-opportunistic, or to non-infectious inflammation (pneumonitis), or tumour formation.

Pneumocystis carinii pneumonia (PCP)

PCP is the initial problem on presentation in more than half of AIDS cases. This is a protozoal infection that only occurs in people who are immuno-compromised. It has an acute mortality rate of up to 35 per cent. The patient presents typically complaining of a dry cough, often of prolonged duration and a sensation of breathlessness. Despite the fact that they have a temperature they rarely complain of fever. Such individuals may not look particularly unwell. Examination may reveal some thrush (candida) in the mouth, fever, and shortness of breath at rest or after minimal exercise. For instance, they may suddenly be unable to talk after climbing a short flight of stairs. There is little to hear on chest examination but an X-ray initially will show a diffuse shadowing. If blood samples are taken to measure blood gases, then blood oxygen may be very low. The patient may look blue around the lips (cyanosis). Alternatively, such patients may present only with a chronic cough and increasing shortness of breath on exertion. The chest X-ray may be normal and the only clue may be the reduced oxygen content of the blood.

Table 4.2 Drugs-related and HIV-related problems

Symptom	*Drug-related**	*HIV-related*
Shortness of breath	Heroin-precipitated asthma, bacterial pneumonia, endocarditis, chronic bronchitis	Pneumocystis pneumonia (PCP), TB
Cough	Bacterial pneumonia, endocarditis, chronic bronchitis.	Pneumocystis pneumonia (PCP), TB
Cyanosis	Bacterial pneumonia, endocarditis, chronic bronchitis	Pneumocystis pneumonia (PCP)
Fever	Injection abscess, septicaemia, pneumonia, endocarditis	Pneumocystis pneumonia (PCP), TB
Rash – small blood spots:	Septicaemia, endocarditis	Thrombocytopenia
– bruises at injection site:	Leakage from injection, arterial injection	Thrombocytopenia
– itchy spots:	Formication associated with amphetamines or cocaine	Allergy, seborrhoeic dermatitis
Abscesses	Missing injection, leakage from injection (especially barbiturates & crushed tablets), infected injection material	Susceptibility to bacterial infection
Sores around mouth	Poor diet, nasal ulceration from snorting cocaine	Chronic cold sores (herpes)
Sore mouth	Poor diet	Cold sores, thrush, oral leukoplakia
Weight loss	Poor diet, anorexic effect of amphetamines or cocaine	CDC IVa, TB, other infections
Vomiting	Opiate withdrawal, septicaemia	Infection, gastric irritation, side-effect of treatment
Diarrhoea	Opiate withdrawal	Cryptosporidiosis
Flu-like symptoms	Opiate withdrawal, septicaemia, endocarditis	CDC III/IVa
Sweating	Opiate withdrawal, septicaemia	CDC III/IVa, TB
Night sweats	Insufficient opiate cover	CDC III/IVa
Loss of vision	Endocarditis, local injection, candida infection of eye	Cytomegalovirus (CMV infection)

Confusion	Drug use, pneumonia, endocarditis, meningitis	Meningitis, toxoplasmosis etc.
Fits/episodic loss of consciousness	Drug overdose, bacterial meningitis, withdrawal (alcohol, barbiturates, benzodiazepines), cocaine-induced fit	Meningitis, toxoplasmosis etc.
Paralysis	Nerve damage from injection	CDC III/IVa

* The term 'drug-related' is used broadly to include those problems associated with route of administration.

Patients with cytomegalovirus (a virus from the herpes family) or fungal pneumonia may have a similar presentation. In addition, the risks of systemic infection resulting from contaminants entering during injecting (such as from contamination with candida – see p.39) are markedly greater in the immunocompromised patient. Patients with a bacterial pneumonia may have a more marked fever with a productive cough and chest pain on coughing.

Tuberculosis

Mycobacterium tuberculosis (TB) infection is more common in the drug-taking population. A recent study from New York (Selwyn *et al.* 1989) found laboratory evidence that similar rates of infection with TB occurred in HIV seronegative and seropositive drug misusers (13 per cent and 11 per cent respectively over 22 months); but that active clinical TB only developed in the HIV-seropositive drug misusers (4 per cent). It may occur at an earlier stage of HIV disease and be particularly difficult to diagnose (see Chapter 24). Recent work has suggested TB infection may be a possible co-factor for HIV progression. Unusual forms of the TB bacillus such as mycobacterium avium complex or mycobacterium kansasii also occur in the later stages of HIV disease more frequently and are important complications.

Bacterial pneumonia

Conventional pneumonia is also commoner in HIV patients. Recurrent bacterial infections are particularly problematic in the injecting drug-using population. This may be due to the combination of injecting practices, exposure to various drugs including alcohol and an impaired antibody response. These infections respond well to appropriate antibiotic treatment, although higher doses and/or longer duration of treatment may be required.

Other lung complications

Kaposi's sarcoma, lymphoid interstitial pneumonia are particular non-infectious complications which may affect the lungs.

Central Nervous System (CNS)

Peripheral nerve damage

HIV can cause a wide range of neurological disorders. Neuropathological abnormalities have been found in 75 to 80 per cent of people who die of AIDS. Considerable attention has recently been paid to the particular affinity of HIV for nerve tissue (see Chapter 5). This may involve individual nerves with resultant nerve palsies or paralysis (especially the facial nerve) or may involve the spinal cord giving rise to weakness or paralysis at lower levels of the body.

Central CNS involvement

More general CNS involvement may give rise to HIV encephalopathy or AIDS dementia. Patients typically complain of forgetfulness, slowness of thought, lack of concentration and difficulties with problem-solving. The diagnosis of AIDS dementia is complicated when the patient is simultaneously taking psychoactive drugs which may themselves be responsible for the symptomatology; the diagnosis should be made only after excluding the possibility of treatable focal opportunistic infections such as cerebral toxoplasmosis, cytomegalovirus and cryptococcus meningitis and mycobacterium tuberculosis or candida albicans.

Gastrointestinal system

The gut is a frequent and symptomatically very troublesome site of involvement. The drug taker may already have poor dental hygiene giving rise to dental abscesses which may be masked by the analgesic drugs being used. Referral to a dental surgeon is advisable. The commonest problem is oral thrush (candida albicans) which may extend from the mouth (oral candidiasis) into the gullet (oesophageal candidiasis) causing difficulty in swallowing. Herpes simplex or cytomegalovirus may cause ulceration on the lips or in the mouth. If the patient complains of difficulty in swallowing, it may be necessary to examine and take a sample (biopsy) from the oesophagus through an endoscope to differentiate between candida, herpes or CMV inflammation.

Oral hairy leukoplakia (OHL) is a condition which is rarely seen outside HIV disease and which results in white plaques on the side of the tongue, and is associated with the Epstein-Barr virus (the virus which causes glandular fever). Aphthous ulcers also occur and may be deep and troublesome.

Diarrhoea is a recurring problem in 70 per cent of patients with active HIV disease. This may be accompanied by weight loss and malabsorption of ingested food. Sometimes this may be infective in origin and this may be determined by repeated stool culture.

Cryptosporidium muris (condition: cryptosporidiosis) causes an explosive, watery diarrhoea with abdominal pain, wasting and severe weight loss. Untreated infection can lead to long-term diarrhoea and malabsorption. Isospora belli is a related organism and gives rise to a similar clinical picture; it is of particular interest in the drug-taking population (see Chapter 24).

Giardia lamblia (condition: giardiasis) is a protozoan infection of sudden onset involving the small bowel and causing diarrhoea with foul-smelling stools and malabsorption. Amoebasis may also occur.

Salmonella, shigella and campylobacter are bacterial infections of the gut that may be severe in immuno-compromised patients and may give rise to septicaemia.

Tumour involvement of the bowel with Kaposi's sarcoma is extremely unusual in the heterosexual drug-using population.

Liver

Many injecting drug takers display abnormalities of liver function tests. Up to 12 per cent become chronic carriers of hepatitis B surface antigen and are able to transmit hepatitis B Virus (HBV) to others. Hepatitis Delta Virus (HDV) may be superimposed on hepatitis B infection and will result in a more severe and progressive liver cirrhosis. Delta Virus has most frequently been found in patients with haemophilia and in injecting drug users. The influence of HIV infection on the course of this illness is unclear.

The risk-taking behaviour involved in exposure to the virus is such that serious consideration should be given to offering hepatitis B vaccine to all injecting drug users (and possibly their sexual partners also). Other opportunistic infections such as mycobacterium avium-intracellulare, cytomegalovirus and cryptococcus neoformans may sometimes cause hepatitis.

Skin

Skin problems are very important from the symptomatic point of view and may cause great distress to the patient. They may in some instances be the first indication of the presence of HIV infection and in other cases the most obvious sign of the progression of the disease. They frequently involve the face and cause distress on cosmetic grounds alone. In seborrhoeic dermatitis, there may be a scaling of skin – particularly around the nose, mouth, eyebrows and scalp margins. Folliculitis is a common, severely itchy rash in hair areas, on the forehead, neck, limbs and shoulders. Psoriasis and xeroderma (dry skin) also occur.

Herpes simplex, which is commonly dormant in the area around the mouth in the general population, may reactivate and cause painful skin and mouth lesions with progression of the disease. Herpes zoster or shingles may also occur or recur. (Oral hairy leukoplakia has been described on p.47.)

As the disease progresses, cellulitis, thrombophlebitis and subcutaneous abscesses are particular problems in the injecting drug users, even those with good sterile technique.

Genito-urinary system

Like all others at risk from HIV, drug users should be screened for sexually transmitted disease. Drug workers, while excelling in counselling on drug use, do not fare so well in talking about sexual practices. It is very important to emphasise the risks involved in unprotected sex (France *et al.* 1988). A small but important group of drug users may be involved in homosexual or heterosexual prostitution. Their risk for contracting or transmitting HIV through unprotected sex is high and needs to be addressed directly.

HIV-positive patients with herpetic oral ulceration may also have genital or anal ulceration. This should be routinely inquired about. HIV-negative patients with genital ulceration appear to be at higher risk from HIV infection and should be counselled about prevention (Piot and Laga 1989). Along with encouraging the use of barriers/contraceptives to protect against infection, family planning advice should be available.

Constitutional symptoms

Fever and weight loss are two major features of the progression of the disease. Weight loss may occur due to poor appetite, difficulty in swallowing or to malabsorption. However, weight loss is also a common feature of amphetamine or cocaine use (due in part to their appetite-suppressing effect), and also frequently occurs during heavy opiate use. Fatigue may also occur. The combination of these symptoms and unusual infections may be the first indication of illness. An awareness of these signs and symptoms may help to detect serious underlying opportunistic infections at an early stage when treatment will be easier and more effective.

MANAGEMENT

As with other HIV risk groups, management is based on the reduction in the extent of initial infection, reduction of the progression to AIDS, and specific treatment directed against HIV. The measures to prevent spread and to reduce possible progression to AIDS are much the same.

As far as the management of drug misuse is concerned, wherever possible one should promote abstinence from opiates and other such drugs because these drugs are immunosuppressive and may reduce resistance to infection. However, if this is not an achievable short-term goal then the use of oral opiate substitute drugs (such as oral methadone) to reduce injectable drug use should be considered (see Chapters 13 and 19). If the drug taker is continuing to inject regularly or even occasionally, then attention must be paid to ensuring that information is given on ways of reducing the risks of HIV infection or transmission. This may be through the provision of information on cleaning needles and syringes, and/or where to obtain clean equipment (see Chapters 14 and 20).

It is theoretically possible that further infection with HIV might occur by sex or needle sharing. Evidence from blood transfusion cases suggests that total dose is important as far as speed of progression is concerned. There is also evidence that continued injecting increases the rate of decline of T4 lymphocytes, aggravated by the injection of impure material into the circulation, which is known to stimulate the immune system. A stimulated immune system seems to promote HIV multiplication. In addition, the use of unsterile equipment leaves the patient open to further bacterial and viral infections: this might well be the drug user's equivalent of a sexually transmitted disease in homosexuals which is believed to hasten the onset of HIV illness.

Treatment with zidovudine (AZT)

Zidovudine has been shown to increase survival and lessen the morbidity of patients with AIDS and ARC. However, because 60 to 70 per cent of zidovudine is metabolised via liver glucoronidation, the potential for a number of drug interactions is considerable. The early toxicity studies noted an association between neutropenia and concurrent paracetamol ingestion. More recently, dosage regimes of 250mg four times daily have been used and are more acceptable to patients, with close monitoring for toxicity in a highly motivated patient group. Patients may feel nauseous and suffer headaches – especially during the early weeks of treatment – and frequent blood tests are required to look for any associated drop in the red or white blood cell counts. Consequently, concerns have been voiced as to whether it is possible to treat ongoing drug misusers with zidovudine. However, preliminary experience with zidovudine and current drug misusers suggests that it is possible, although there are of course problems. There have not yet been any untoward reactions with benzodiazepines, opiates, cannabis or alcohol (cocaine use is rare in the study groups). One major problem, by comparison with homosexuals, is the relatively poor attendance; however, there was little difference in attendance between ex-users, those on oral methadone or those still injecting. The most reliable patients (perhaps not surprisingly) were those receiving opiate prescription at the same time as zidovudine (Cowan and Brettle 1989).

Zidovudine therapy presents a number of practical issues which are more specific to injecting drug users. Currently, because of the unknown effect of zidovudine upon the foetus, termination may be advisable in the case of pregnancy. Whilst in theory zidovudine might actually reduce the chance of infection in the foetus, it is known to interfere with DNA synthesis and could result in foetal damage.

The improvement in health induced by zidovudine may result in individuals feeling well enough to recommence former drug-taking ways. Injection of drugs will continue to occur in patients on zidovudine treatment and this situation emphasises the importance of repeating harm-minimisation messages.

Lastly, the original four-hourly regime may be impracticable for the life-style of many drug users. There is now evidence appearing that this routine may not be necessary. A six- to eight-hourly regime based on meal times appears satisfactory. The major objective must be to get the patients to take the daily dose and not to worry too much about exact timings.

CONCLUSION

All drug workers must become HIV-cognisant and HIV-competent. Routine regular contact with drug users should include running through a health checklist (such as in Table 4.3) to increase early detection of disease progression. It seems likely that tomorrow's drug worker will need to be as comfortable with checking for oral thrush and taking a blood sample as with today's comfortable areas of considering prescribing options and looking for relapse precipitants.

What does the future hold in store? Until we better understand the natural history of drug users with HIV and the factors affecting progression, management strategies will be difficult to develop. For instance, it was initially thought that pregnancy was detrimental to the health of HIV-positive women. However, this is now uncertain since the initial reports were influenced by selection bias. Gender may well be something that must be allowed for in assessing progression: in New York City, females seem less susceptible; in Scotland, they seem more susceptible in the early stages. Gender may also affect presentation – for example, immuno-compromised women have an increased risk of cervical cancer.

Table 4.3 Health checklist

Chest
Shortness of breath with or without dry cough, with or without fever (especially sudden onset)
Eyes
Blurred vision; sensitivity to light (photophobia)
Brain
Headache; epileptic fits of recent onset; weakness; recent onset of memory loss or confusion

Any of the above should be reasons for considering urgent assessment of possible HIV disease.

Systemic symptoms
Fatigue; loss of energy; night sweats; swollen lymph nodes, especially around head and neck
Mouth
Ulcers and sores; white deposits of candida; difficulty swallowing
Gut
Diarrhoea; recent loss of weight; loss of appetite; anal warts or ulcers
Skin
Dry skin; seborrhoeic dermatitis; eczema; herpes simplex; shingles; pigmented lesions of Kaposi's sarcoma (more common in HIV-positive homosexuals)
Ear, nose and throat
Sinusitis; catarrh; ear infections

Further work is needed to determine whether continued drug use by injection, orally or by inhalation has an influence on outcome and whether the prescribing of substitute drugs results in any durable change in risk-taking behaviour or has an effect on HIV disease progression. The importance of bacterial infections must not be overlooked; in New York City, there are as many HIV-positive injectors who die from bacterial pneumonia as from AIDS (see Chapter 24). Thus, this susceptibility of bacterial infections needs to be considered.

Lastly, treatment regimes for HIV-positive drug users must take into account continued drug use. For instance, complex schedules, the need for frequent blood tests, a lack of venous access or drug interactions might all make a particular treatment impossible in certain situations, and will certainly force consideration of combined treatment approaches in which both the drug problem and the HIV disease are treated simultaneously.

REFERENCES

Cowan, F.M. and Brettle, R.P. (1989) 'Use of zidovudine for drug misusers infected with HIV', *Journal of Infection* 18 (supplement 1: 59–66.

Des Jarlais, D.C., Wish, E., Friedman, S.R., Stoneburner, R. *et al.* (1987) 'Intravenous drug use and the heterosexual transmission of the Human Immunodeficiency Virus: current trends in New York City', *New York State Journal of Medicine*, May: 283–6.

France, A.J., Skidmore, C.A. and Robertson, J.R. (1988) 'Heterosexual spread of HIV in Edinburgh', *British Medical Journal* 296: 526–9.

Hay, R.J. (1986) 'Systemic candidiasis in heroin addicts', *British Medical Journal*, 292: 1096.

Lifson, A.R., Rutherford, G.W. and Jaffe, H.W. (1988) 'The natural history of Human Immunodeficiency Virus infection', *Journal of Infectious Diseases* 158(6): 1360–7.

Piot, P. and Laga, M. (1989) 'Genital ulcers, other sexually transmitted diseases, and the sexual transmission of HIV', *British Medical Journal*, 298: 623–4.

Selwyn, P.A., Hartel, D., Lewis, V.A., Schoenbaum, E.E., Vermund, S.H., Klein, R.S., Walker, A.T. and Friedland, G.H. (1989) 'A prospective study of the risk of tuberculosis among intravenous drug users with Human Immunodeficiency Virus infection', *New England Journal of Medicine* 320: 545–50.

Chapter Five

NEUROPSYCHIATRIC COMPLICATIONS OF HIV INFECTION

MASSIMO RICCIO AND DAVID HAWKINS

It is difficult to conceive of any other medical event in recent history which has created as much public and private fear as AIDS. From the very first diagnosis of HIV antibody positivity, people have to cope not only with knowledge of their infection but also with the burden of stress arising from the reactions of society, family and friends. It is hardly surprising, therefore, that mental health issues form an integral part of HIV infection, in terms of both symptomatology and treatment.

The majority of psychiatric manifestations in HIV-seropositive individuals arise from the stresses related to knowledge of the infection. These lead most to adjustment reactions and mild and transitory affective responses, such as free-floating anxiety and reactive depression. A minority of people may present with more severe psychiatric symptoms, such as major mood disturbances, in the form of acute anxiety states, panic attacks or severe depression, and psychotic states. It is important to distinguish in this context the more psychological reactions to the infection just described, from the symptoms arising out of the Central Nervous System (CNS) involvement. The latter can be seen in patients with HIV disease, and take the form of acute confusional states and chronic impairment of intellectual functioning leading to dementia.

Although most of the knowledge to date on the neuropsychiatric complications of HIV infection stems from observations in populations of homosexual men, it is reasonable to infer that much of this will also apply to a population of drug users. Historically, injecting drug users and homosexual men have been stigmatised on the basis of social prejudices concerning their lifestyle. In addition, since HIV is acquired primarily through sexual contact or the injection of drugs and because both of these activities may incur moral judgements, some HIV-positive drug users may feel blamed for the illness. Furthermore, the diagnosis of HIV seropositivity and AIDS may come to shatter a belief of immortality developed by drug users during their sustained risky life-styles, thus potentially leading to feelings of loss of control.

In this chapter we shall try to review the present state of knowledge of the neuropsychiatric complications of HIV infection and speculate on the likely impact of these for the management of drug users found to be HIV positive.

DISTRESS OF DIAGNOSIS

Even the decision to request an HIV test is likely to raise a number of conflicts. Subsequently, the impact of the diagnosis of HIV seropositivity often leads to expressions of anxiety, despair, grief, guilt and depression. These reactions are common to many life events and diseases, but in the case of HIV infection are often aggravated by the collapse of the patient's social network, the stigma attached to the infection, the threat to financial security, relationships, self-esteem, independence, health and eventually life itself.

A careful assessment of those people who may be more at risk of developing severe psychological distress following diagnosis should be made at the time of pre-test counselling. It is important to make sure that the user is properly counselled as to the meaning of the antibody test and its results, positive or negative. In particular an exploration of support systems should be undertaken even though these may already have been disrupted by the drug user's previous anti-social behaviour.

Post-test counselling for patients found to be HIV seropositive should contain elements of information-giving, expression of feelings, and support. Anxiety linked to a recent diagnosis of positivity has often a common denominator in the uncertainty thrown into the patient's life. This should be dealt with by providing clarification of the issues leading to the uncertainty in the form of straight talk and fact-giving. Some patients may be overwhelmed by emotion, and may engage in life-threatening behaviour. Thus, drug users may return to chaotic drug-taking, sexual behaviour and at times suicidal behaviour.

PSYCHIATRIC COMPLICATIONS IN ASYMPTOMATIC AND SYMPTOMATIC HIV DISEASE

Not surprisingly, psychological distress varies with the changes in the clinical stages of the disease. People with AIDS Related Complex (ARC), who may have moderate to severe physical symptoms but do not have the 'terminal' diagnosis of AIDS, have been shown to have higher levels of psychological distress than people who are still asymptomatic or people with AIDS (Holland and Tross 1985). This is thought to be due to their uncertain prognosis. Some of these patients may present with moderate anxiety states and recurrent panic attacks and sleep disturbance is common (Catalan 1988).

In the early stages it may be difficult to distinguish depression and anxiety from the early symptoms of HIV disease. Features common to all three conditions are weight loss, forgetfulness, loss of concentration, loss of energy and loss of appetite. Pathological anxiety may affect the patient's ability to cope with daily tasks, such as work and relationships. Depression may also be the presenting symptom of CNS involvement either by HIV itself or by secondary opportunistic infections or tumours. A useful pointer to the diagnosis of a major depressive illness in these patients is indicated by the presence of a severe and persistent depressed mood, with little or no variation. In addition, hopelessness about the future, tearfulness, overwhelming feelings of guilt and self-blame and at times suicidal ideation may be present. For injecting drug users the problem may be further compounded by a pre-morbid tendency to depression and self-harm.

Counselling as outlined above remains a first-line approach, and in cases of severe anxiety and depressive states it may be appropriate to institute more specific treatment approaches, such as anxiety-management techniques. Anti-depressant drugs should be used in cases of severe depression. HIV infection itself does not preclude the use of psychotropic medication where appropriate, despite the fact that these patients do have a tendency to develop more frequent side-effects to medication. Admission to a psychiatric unit may be needed when the patient is suicidal. Patients with

AIDS often view their suicidal ideation and intent as reasonable, considering the social stigma of the disease and its progressive and ultimately fatal course. However, it is important not to accept this explanation in the presence of a depressive illness and every effort should be made to treat the depression appropriately.

PSYCHIATRIC PROBLEMS IN PEOPLE WITH AIDS

The diagnosis of AIDS leads to a range of psychological reactions, both normal and abnormal, which may be comparable to those encountered in other serious medical conditions. Depression, sadness, suicidal ideas, guilt with a perception of illness as retribution, social isolation, fear about the disease and about what the future holds are often seen. In addition the diagnosis often leads to stressful changes in life-style, a sense of loss, and – in the case of Kaposi's sarcoma of the skin – stigmata, which may all contribute to the psychological make-up of people with AIDS. Associated declining physical and at times mental ability add to the psychological distress. It is at this stage that the most severe psychological and psychiatric manifestations are seen, such as major depression or psychoses.

In the case of injecting drug users the impact of diagnosis may be compounded by the rejections of health care staff, such as being deemed unsuitable for admission to treatment programmes.

STRESS, DEPRESSION AND IMMUNITY

Evidence from both animal and human studies suggests a link between stress, depression and immune function. These studies seem to link psychological distress with disease progression and treatment outcome. A few studies have looked at the relationship between psychological states and disease outcome in human patients with diseases involving the immune system. However, insufficient attention is being paid to the relationship between psychological and immunological variables and how they relate to HIV disease outcome. Although AIDS is widely thought by the lay public and professional community to be an invariably fatal disease, some individuals with AIDS remain alive and well longer than others. It is possible to speculate, therefore, that psychological factors may play a role in prolonging survival (Temoshok 1988).

The complex interaction between psychological, behavioural and immunological variables is further compounded in a population of injecting drug users by the known action of the drugs on the immune system. Several studies have reported on the immunomodulatory effects of alcohol, cocaine and opiates (Donahoe and Falek, 1988). In addition, data from Edinburgh (Cowan *et al.* 1989) and New York City (Des Jarlais *et al.* 1985) seems to support the generally held view that injectable street drugs have a negative effect on physical health and a specific immune-suppressive action when compared to abstinence and oral methadone.

Despite the need for further research into this interesting field it is nevertheless clear that health professionals should be aware of the likely association between HIV infection and psychological distress and its likely negative influence on immune function, in order to set up interventions aimed at preventing such distress and alleviating it when present.

HIV INFECTION AND THE CENTRAL NERVOUS SYSTEM

HIV-related dementia

Neurological and neuropsychiatric complications form an integral part of HIV disease. HIV has been demonstrated to be present in the CNS and up to 75 to 80 per cent of people who die of AIDS have been shown to have neuropathological findings. CNS complications of HIV disease can occur either as a direct action of HIV itself or through the development of opportunistic infections or tumours of the brain secondary to the immune suppression.

People with HIV disease may develop symptoms suggestive of organic brain disease leading to dementia. Individuals with HIV-related dementia typically complain of forgetfulness, slowness of thought, lack of concentration, difficulties with problem solving. They may appear withdrawn, apathetic and in some cases there is a typically neurological component in the form of movement disorders. A clinical examination of these patients will demonstrate lack of attention, psychomotor slowing, impaired retrieval of information and concentration. In addition, focal or generalised neurological problems may be revealed (Riccio and Thompson 1987).

Formal neuropsychological testing may show abnormalities including reduced problem-solving ability, visual–spatial deficits, learning difficulties and poor short- and medium-term memory (Riccio *et al.* 1988). As these symptoms are not specific to HIV dementia but are mostly found in generalised encephalopathies, a diagnosis of HIV dementia should be made only after careful exclusion, by laboratory and radiographic means, of other causes of CNS involvement which may be treatable. The finding of abnormalities in the cerebral spinal fluid including specific anti-HIV antibodies locally produced is a relatively non-specific finding, as it can occur in neurologically and neuropsychologically normal HIV-infected people (McArthur 1987).

There are no available data on the incidence of dementia in people with HIV disease, although clinical experience suggests that the more severe forms of dementia are normally seen in the later stages of HIV disease and that the emergence of clinically evident dementia is a sign of poor prognosis, usually occurring in the last few weeks or months of life. Point prevalence of dementia in people with HIV disease has been said to range between 8 and 16 per cent (McArthur 1987). The variation in prevalence data in the different studies may be the result of factors such as sample selection, regional variations in populations and differences in diagnostic criteria and techniques used. In addition, different neurotropism in HIV strains and coexisting infections may play a role.

There are no known risk factors associated with the development of dementia in people with HIV infection. In particular, it is not yet known whether the finding of mild or subclinical neuropsychological abnormalities in asymptomatic seropositives is associated with later development of dementia. Whether different routes of infection are involved in different manifestations or courses of dementia is yet to be determined, but there is some evidence that secondary opportunistic infections of the CNS are commoner in injecting drug users when compared to homosexual men (Levy *et al.* 1988).

Neuropsychological abnormalities without dementia

HIV-infected individuals with clinically evident dementia will be diagnosed as having AIDS under the current Centers for Disease Control classification (see Chapter 4). However, cognitive or behavioural problems may occur in people in Group I, II, III and IV (non-AIDS), i.e. across the full spectrum of degree of clinical expression.

These patients may complain of difficulties with concentration, memory, speech and language, sometimes associated with headaches, incoordination, weakness and apathy. Neuropsychological testing may show problems in the complex perceptual, motor, performance and abstracting abilities, motor slowing and at times poor performance on tests of learning and recall. These abnormalities are usually mild and are not sufficient to establish a diagnosis of dementia and the people affected are usually able to continue to lead an independent life-style (World Health Organization 1988).

The abnormalities described, detected by history and neuropsychological testing are non-specific and may be due to functional psychiatric disorders such as anxiety and depressive states, or other factors influencing brain function such as other infections including syphilis, metabolic disturbances or head injuries. In the case of drug users we are again faced with the problem of differentiating the effect of the substance of abuse itself on brain function from HIV-related symptomatology.

Different studies of neuropsychological testing of HIV-seropositive individuals report differing rates of abnormalities varying from 0 to 44 per cent in HIV-seropositive, asymptomatic individuals and from 0 to 54 per cent in people with ARC (Catalan 1988). The wide variations reported by different researchers may be accounted for by the same factors used to explain the variability in the incidence rate of HIV-related dementia. In trying to understand the meaning and prognostic value of such findings it is important to remember that most of the data stem from preliminary reports of longitudinal follow-up studies of selected populations of homosexual men. Some studies also report a high number of abnormalities, compared to the published norms for the test used, in HIV-negative controls (Catalan 1988). When comparing actual performance on individual neuropsychological tests, regardless of cut-offs determined by published population norms, some studies report HIV-positive subjects performing worse than HIV-negative controls and others report no difference (Catalan, 1988; Riccio *et al.* 1988). The meaning of such abnormalities will therefore become clearer only on completion of the current longitudinal studies and by controlling appropriately for such factors as mood states, previous medical and psychiatric history, and current and past abuse of drugs including alcohol.

Given the methodological difficulty of carrying out a well-controlled longitudinal study of neuropsychological testing in drug users, it is hardly surprising that most of the data available to date relate to populations of homosexual men and not specifically to drug users. However, one study that has looked at 211 drug users on a methadone programme found evidence of impaired performance on some of the neuropsychological tests in the HIV seropositives compared to the seronegatives (Silberstein *et al.* 1987).

IMPLICATIONS FOR MANAGEMENT OF INJECTING DRUG USERS

The combination of injecting drug use and HIV infection compounds problems encountered in the treatment of both conditions. Treatment of drug dependence will have to take account of the likely psychological, neuropsychiatric and physical consequences of HIV infection. From a neuropsychiatric point of view, the manifestations encountered in HIV infection are non-specific. It is therefore difficult to disentangle them from similar manifestations caused by the use of drugs or pre-morbid traits. Although the more functionally psychiatric accompaniments of HIV infection can successfully be dealt with by an understanding and non-judgemental approach within existing addiction treatment facilities, it is possible that problems may be encountered with the emergence of more specific CNS involvement. In the treatment setting, such people may require the provision of less challenging treatment approaches for their drug use. This may require professionals to modify existing regimes, whilst continuing to encourage the patient towards abandoning injecting behaviours. Highly confrontational and restrictive approaches may need to be replaced by more supportive and individually tailored programmes with greater emphasis on physical and psychiatric care. These may be difficult to set up within existing treatment programmes where the establishment of 'special' rules may be seen as detrimental to the overall treatment philosophy of the community.

Unfortunately, there is no one single answer to the problem; nevertheless, it is possible that solutions may be found by the setting up of a range of services aimed at drug users with varying needs according to their HIV status. In any case it is important to tackle the problem, rather than to discount it and set the ground for yet one more rejection at the expense of the individual with HIV infection and society.

On the basis of our current knowledge there is no evidence that major neuropsychiatric complications are associated with sero-positive status, and drug dependence rehabilitation programmes will only need to be aware that there may be a minority of people at later stages of HIV disease who may be cognitively impaired and for whom a more conservative approach may be indicated. It is, however, possible that this picture may change with time and with the development of more effective anti-HIV treatments.

REFERENCES

Catalan, J. (1988) 'Psychosocial and neuropsychiatric aspects of HIV infection: review of their extent and implications for psychiatry', *Journal of Psychosomatic Research* 32(3): 237–48.

Cowan, F.M., Jones, G., Bingham, J. and others (1989) 'Use of zidovudine for drug misusers infected with HIV', *Journal of Infections* 18(1): 59–66.

Des Jarlais, D.C., Friedman, S.R., Hopkins, W. (1985) 'Risk reduction for the Acquired Immunodeficiency Syndrome among intravenous drug users', *Annals of Internal Medicine* 103: 755–9.

Donahoe, R.M. and Falek, A. (1988) 'Neuroimmunomodulation by opiates and other drugs of abuse: relationship to HIV infection and AIDS', in T.P. Bridge *et al.* (eds) *Psychological, Neuropsychiatric and Substance Abuse Aspects of AIDS*, New York: Raven Press.

Holland, J.C. and Tross, S. (1985) 'The psychosocial and neuropsychiatric sequelae of the Immunodeficiency Syndrome and related disorders', *Annals of Internal Medicine* 103: 760–4.

Levy, R.M., Janssen, R.S., Bush, T.J. *et al.* (1988) 'Neuroepidemiology of Acquired Immunodeficiency Syndrome', *Journal of Acquired Immunodeficiency Syndromes* 1: 31–40.

McArthur, J.C. (1987) 'Neurologic manifestations of AIDS', *Medicine* 66(6): 407–37.

Riccio, M. and Thompson, C. (1987) 'AIDS dementia', *British Journal of Hospital Medicine* 38(1): 11.

Riccio, M., Hawkins, D., Wilson, B. *et al* (1988) 'Neuropsychiatric manifestations of early HIV disease', paper presented at the 4th International Conference on AIDS, Stockholm, Sweden.

Silberstein, C.H., McKegney, F.P., O'Dowd, M. *et al.* (1987) 'A prospective longitudinal study of neuropsychological and psychosocial factors in asymptomatic individuals at risk for HTLV III/LAV infection in a methadone programme: preliminary findings', *International Journal of Neurosciences* 32: 669–76.

Temoshok, L. (1988) 'Psychoimmunology and AIDS', in T.P. Bridge *et al.* (eds) *Psychological, Neuropsychiatric and Substance Abuse Aspects of AIDS*, New York: Raven Press.

World Health Organization (1988) *Global Programme on AIDS. Report of the Consultation on the Neuropsychiatric Aspects of HIV Infection*, Geneva: World Health Organization.

Part Three

UNDERSTANDING THE EPIDEMIC

Chapter Six

DRUG-USING TRENDS AND HIV RISK BEHAVIOUR

ROBERT POWER

The prime objective of this chapter is a simple one: to show the diversity of patterns of drug use and to identify the ways in which they influence HIV-related risk behaviour. Trends in drug use, along with the consumers themselves and behaviours associated with the risk of HIV infection, are situated in time and place, and operate according to three sets of shifting paradigms: the social; the political; and the personal.

At the social level, swings in the illicit drug market and regional and cultural variations will influence drug-using patterns and routes of administration. At the political level, varying government attitudes towards illicit drugs will determine the judicial and treatment policy climate in which drug use takes place. At the personal level, individuals at different stages of their drug-using careers will make decisions about their own drug use. These decisions will cover issues such as: the types, frequency and quantities of drugs to be consumed; the favoured route of administration; and the strategies to be adopted to endeavour to control such use.

None of the above are static, and all interrelate in determining any individual's level of risk behaviour in relation to HIV infection. Additionally, drug users (like everyone else) are at risk of HIV infection if they fail to practise safer sex. Presently, this issue will be addressed in the specific context of the drug user, but a prior task is to examine patterns of drug use.

PATTERNS OF USE, AND SOCIETAL AND REGIONAL DIVERSITY

There is considerable variation between individual countries in the history and patterns of drug use. The Pompidou Group (1987) has compared and contrasted the history, treatment policy, legislation and contemporary scenario of illicit drug use across seven European cities. For instance, in Amsterdam heroin superseded opium and amphetamines when it was introduced by Vietnam veterans in the early 1970s. The late 1980s witnessed a further swing, with polydrug use and cocaine gaining in popularity and heroin use declining. In Dublin, a Ministry of Health report of the early 1970s highlighted a continued trend in polydrug use, especially amphetamines, barbiturates, and tranquillisers, but found no evidence of heroin use. It was not until the 1980s that heroin use was identified in numbers sufficient to cause official concern and comment. Meanwhile, the Paris drug scene up to 1973 was dominated by psychedelic products such as cannabis and LSD. Although heroin was available, the market was disorganised, and the small number of users were closely knit. Some years later, in the wake of the infamous 'French Connection', heroin of Asian origin found its way to Paris via Marseilles, with an increase in use of the drug in the late 1970s and early 1980s. The experience of Stockholm is peculiar in that the popularity of amphetamines has continued almost uninterrupted ever since the introduction of Phenedrin and Benzedrine in the late 1930s, with 1942 witnessing the licit and illicit consumption of six million tablets. Successive decades brought love affairs with a range of drugs – LSD, cannabis and heroin – but throughout, the Swedes have maintained their fidelity to 'speed'. Recent estimates suggest that 80 per cent of regular drug injectors use amphetamines as their drug of choice, compared with only 30 per cent favouring opiates (mainly heroin). Across the Atlantic in the USA, the recent upsurge in cocaine use and especially the smoking of 'crack', along with the popularity of designer drugs, represents an emerging trend yet to be observed on anything like the same scale in Europe.

Not surprisingly, differences in patterns of drug use occur within, as well as between, countries. In specific areas of the north of England, the preference for amphetamines (and notably in our context, the injecting of amphetamines) contrasted with the media and political emphasis placed on the highly visible heroin use in major cities such as London and Liverpool. A number of other social factors determine the types of drugs that are available and the way in which they are used. The world's pharmaceutical industries have a partial responsibility for the unfolding of trends in illicit drug use, in that many mind-altering pharmaceutical products eventually find a niche in the illicit market. At the same time, changes in the price, type and quality of drugs being offered on the illicit market will not only influence the trends in drug use (heroin yesterday, 'crack' and Ecstasy tomorrow), but also the way in which they are administered. For instance, there are occasions when the heroin on the market literally disappears in a puff of smoke when ignited, prompting some to turn from smoking to injecting. Alternatively, some heroin (particularly 'brown' heroin from Iran and Pakistan) contains many impurities, is specifically prepared for smoking and requires arduous purification to render it suitable for injecting. In such instances, injectors revert, albeit temporarily, to smoking (see, for example, Pearson 1987). Recently, the birth (or, more correctly, the reincarnation) of 'crack' has led to a new cohort of smokers amongst the world's drug-using fraternity. In like manner, the designer drugs represent a revival of the oral route of administration amongst illicit users. Clearly, differential patterns of routes of administration are crucial in relation to risk behaviour and are closely linked to trends in drug use.

There are a number of imperatives that determine the preferred route of administration for any particular drug or drug user. Some individuals, like those who restrict their use to cannabis or LSD, will have little or no tradition of injecting drugs within their drug subculture. On the other hand, cultural factors play a part in determining the favoured route of administration. In Holland, the Moluccan and Surinamese ethnic minorities traditionally smoke illicit drugs like cocaine and heroin, with injecting being a rare exception (Wijngaart 1988). Interestingly, a similar cultural taboo against injecting exists amongst the Afro-Caribbean community in Britain, but is not mirrored in the USA, where injecting amongst black drug users is common. In Britain, a number of studies point to the importance of regional and social traditions in determining the dominant route of administration of illicit drugs, especially heroin. In the major cities of Scotland there is an almost exclusive tradition of injecting (see Chapter 9). Some miles south into England, the predominant trend amongst heroin users in the Wirral, throughout most of the 1980s, was to smoke the drug, or 'chase the dragon'. One study found that only 4 per cent of 652 regular heroin users injected as a sole means of administration, compared with 79 per cent who smoked (Parker *et al.* 1988). Another study in the north of England highlighted the influence of established modes of administering drugs (especially amphetamines) in determining the way in which new drugs would be used. So, in an area where injecting was commonplace, cheap heroin – which arrived on the scene in the 1980s – was automatically injected (Pearson 1987; see also Power 1988).

POLITICAL IMPERATIVES AND VARIETY IN TREATMENT OPTIONS

At the political level, decisions and shifts in thinking around treatment and judicial policy have an influence upon drug-using patterns and proclivity towards high-risk behaviour. Most pertinent is the political issue of needle and syringe availability. Varying political reactions to this issue have led to a wide spectrum of responses. In Holland, the liberal approach to drug use has resulted in free availability of injecting equipment (see Chapter 14). In Britain, the response has been more guarded, with some initial ambivalence succeeding the pilot needle-exchange schemes set up in the mid-1980s (see Chapter 20). In the USA, laws prohibiting the possession of drug 'paraphernalia' inhibit the wide availability of sterile injecting equipment.

Such international dissimilarity in practice and policy adds another element to the diversity in patterns of drug use. Drug taking entails more than just the consumption of illicit substances; it incorporates all the activities that drug users engage in to attain their desired goal. For those who inject, one crucial element of the equation is the time, effort, risks, and sometimes money, involved in obtaining sterile injecting equipment. In this context, varying political responses to needle availability can have a direct influence upon differential exposure to high-risk behaviours. Difficulty in obtaining sterile injecting equipment means time is expended in seeking out venues where clean equipment can be obtained and used. Blackmarkets can develop, requiring drug users to raise additional revenue to cover costs, as occurred in New York City in 1987, where 'sets' were sold at between $3 and $5 according to their quality. Where punitive legislation exists, the conflict between the drug-using community and the judiciary is further exacerbated: drug users are unlikely to ensure that they have sterile equipment close to hand if that equipment might be used as evidence in prosecutions.

More generally, government responses to judicial and treatment options have a direct effect upon patterns of drug use. For instance, the Dutch government's decision to make methadone easily accessible, epitomised by the famous methadone buses, meant that drug users were given the opportunity to rationalise their intake of illicit drugs, which in turn has clear ramifications for the overall pattern of drug use (see Chapter 14). Such a non-repressive attitude to the use of illicit drugs is uncommon. In West Germany, methadone plays a very limited part in treatment and comprises only a small part of the illicit market. Therapeutic communities form the main focus of treatment and methadone is only used for limited detoxification, which is strictly monitored. As in Sweden, a strong control policy exists with no distinction being made in law between different classes of drug. Furthermore, in both Sweden and France, legislation exists that can force convicted drug users to undergo treatment for addiction.

So, both legislation and treatment policy influence drug use, and just as there is no universal legislative and treatment paradigm, neither is there one universally applicable pattern of drug misuse. That exposure to treatment itself has an influence upon drug-using trends has been identified by recent work conducted in London (Hartnoll and Power 1989). Two hundred and forty drug users were interviewed in depth: half were in contact with services ('the agency group'), and half were derived from the wider drug-using community, not in contact with drug agencies ('the non-agency group'). Not altogether surprisingly, one impact of entry into treatment was a reduction (at least in the short term) in demand for illicit heroin and a concomitant significant fall in criminal activity. This change was not observed amongst the non-agency group, who remained out of contact with services. Significantly, the study pointed to the impact of agency contact upon patterns of injecting and sharing. Injectors in the non-agency group reported higher incidences of needle sharing than the agency group when first interviewed. This was amplified at the follow-up interview, some three months later, with the non-agency group being more likely than the agency group still to be injecting and sharing and the latter reporting substantial decreases in these activities. Although the switch from heroin to oral methadone had some role to play, the data suggest that whilst injectors remain out of contact with services, they are likely not only to present a different profile of patterns of drug use from those in contact with services, but are also likely to continue to constitute a group associated with high-risk behaviour (see Power *et al.* 1988).

DRUG CAREERS, CONTROL STRATEGIES AND RELATIVE RISKS

A third level that distinguishes patterns of drug use and related levels of risk behaviour, is the dimension of the individual. Some drug users will restrict their consumption to 'soft' drugs like cannabis. Others will concentrate on opiates (such as heroin), or else develop a passion for stimulants (like cocaine and amphetamines). Another group will become polydrug users, consuming a wide range of substances. Within each of these categories some will become more or less physically or psychologically dependent on the drug; many more will use regularly, but in a controlled way, adopting a variety of strategies to ensure that their drug use is kept in check; and others will be recreational or casual users, consuming their chosen substances at selected times, as and when they become available. In addition, few drug-using 'careers' remain static. Some do manage to retain a constant pattern, but many will oscillate in terms of their involvement and entrenchment in the drug subculture and the range of drugs that they consume. A number of factors are important in determining any individual's pattern of drug use at any given time, predominantly: age, individual circumstances and personality, level of involvement and knowledge of the drug subculture, current legislation, treatment options, and drug availability.

Similar principles apply to the highly relevant issue of routes of administration. Some will only ever smoke their drugs, some will use a variety of routes of administration, and some will always inject. As with drug careers, criteria determining route of administration will rely upon a range of factors, which are themselves far from static. Personal circumstances will play a large part in these decisions, having huge ramifications for individual levels of risk behaviour. For example, an individual building up an expensive drug habit may make a purely pragmatic decision to inject the drug, arguing that this method is the most economical and cost-effective way to administer it. Drug users who find themselves in the specific circumstance of imprisonment, where heroin is available but injecting equipment is scarce, may find themselves sharing needles and increasing their risk of HIV infection. Another circumstantial factor that will often determine the pattern of drug use and level of risk of infection is the 'hit or no hit' syndrome. Injectors often report that if they are desperate for drugs and faced with the dilemma of sharing a needle with another user or remaining abstinent, they will take the former option. Some adopt strategies to guard against such a predicament (ranging from hiding away small amounts of drugs to sending rations to themselves through the post). Of course, all such strategies are tentative, liable to be discarded when a local drugs shortage occurs, or when individuals run out of resources. None the less, such strategies certainly represent an attempt to break the cycle of desperation and needle and syringe sharing.

SEX AND DRUGS AND 'CONDOM RUNS'

Although the issue of needle and syringe sharing is of prime concern, there are a number of levels at which drug users' sexual activity is pertinent to the issue of risk behaviour. This relates to the drug effects themselves, the connection between needle and syringe sharing and high-risk sexual behaviour, and prostitution as a means of revenue-raising. Ferguson *et al.*'s (1974) review of the literature makes it clear that although drug effects are influenced by circumstance, environment and individual personalities, evidence does exist to suggest that specific drugs influence sexual behaviour. Stimulants, particularly cocaine and amphetamines, can act as disinhibitors during the sex act. One study reported that intravenous amphetamine users experienced simultaneous erection and heightened sexual excitement on injecting the drug. In general, the reviewers comment, marijuana is the drug most often reported as producing a physiological effect which appears to be disinhibitory, leading to the enhancement of sexual pleasure and creating excitation during sexual activity. Heroin, however, is often identified as the drug resulting in a decrease in the sex drive and thereby inhibiting sexual activity. It is also common for women heroin users to experience irregular menstrual cycles. Now, regarding HIV infection, both these properties of drugs have the potential to lead to high-risk behaviours. An individual heavily intoxicated with a stimulatory drug is in danger of forgoing safe-sex practices due to its disinhibitory effects. At the other end of the spectrum, where heroin has decreased the sex drive and interrupted the menstrual cycle, there is less incentive to use barrier contraception on the infrequent occasions when sexual activity takes place.

Also, there is the link, at the time of the sex act itself, between high-risk sexual practices and substance abuse. Stall *et al.*'s (1986) study of 463 gay men in San Francisco found a strong relationship between the use of drugs and non-compliance with safe-sex practices. Depending on the specific drug involved, men reporting high-risk sexual activity were 2 to 3.5 times more likely to have used drugs during sexual activity than those practising safe sex, and the likelihood of risk behaviour associated with sexual activity was greater if the drug used was an illicit one. At follow-up, it was found that men who were originally in the 'no-risk' group, but who had subsequently become involved in 'high-risk' sexual practices, were twice as likely than those still at no risk to be using alcohol, 'poppers' or marijuana during the sex act, and seven times more likely to be using other drugs. In London, a recent study at a drug clinic noted the connection between high-risk sexual behaviour and high-risk sharing of needles and syringes (Coleman *et al.* 1988). Similarly, Hart *et al.* (1989) point to instances where one sexual partner in a couple would provide injecting equipment to be shared to enhance the sex act. It was also noted that a quarter of the women in their sample reported having exchanged sex for money in the past year, and this is the third factor linking sex, drugs and high risk behaviour in relation to HIV infection.

Incidents have been highlighted by the media of a post-AIDS phenomenon of a two-tier system of prostitution. One price is demanded for sex with the use of a condom, and another, higher, price for unprotected sex. Clearly, the risks of HIV infection both to prostitute and customer are substantially increased when condoms are not used. Much of this information is anecdotal and it will be of interest to monitor the impact of schemes, such as that operating in Manchester, England (nicknamed the 'condom run'), where outreach workers distribute condoms and health education materials to prostitutes on the streets.

CONCLUSION

Patterns of illicit drug use, routes of administration and sexual practices amongst drug users are dependent upon a number of interrelated factors. Most crucially, political, social and personal dimensions will influence trends, with time and place being significant determinants. It is of the utmost importance that those devising interventions aimed at reducing the spread of HIV are aware of the complex issues that link drug use to the propensity towards high-risk behaviours.

REFERENCES

Coleman, R., Curtis, D. and Feinmann, C. (1988) 'Perception of risk of HIV infection by injecting drug users and effects on medical clinic attendance', *British Journal of Addiction*, 83: 1325–30.

Ferguson, P., Lennox, T. and Lettieri, J. (eds.) (1974) *Drugs and Sex*, Maryland: National Institute on Drug Abuse.

Hart, G., Sonnex, C., Petherick, A., Johnson, A., Feinmann, C. and Adler, M. (1989) 'Risk behaviours for HIV infection amongst injecting drug users attending a drug dependency clinic', *British Medical Journal* 298: 1081–3.

Hartnoll, R. and Power, R. (1989) *A Study of Help-seeking and Service Utilisation by Problem Drug Takers*, London: Department of Health (available from ISDD (Institute for the Study of Drug Dependence)).

Parker, H., Bakx, K. and Newcombe, R. (1988) *Living with Heroin*, Milton Keynes: Open University Press.

Pearson, G. (1987) *The New Heroin Users*, London: Blackwell.

Pompidou Group (1987) *Multi-city Study of Drug Misuse in Amsterdam, Dublin, Hamburg, London, Paris, Rome and Stockholm*, Strasbourg: Council of Europe.

Power, R. (1988) 'The influence of AIDS upon patterns of intravenous use – syringe and needle sharing – among illicit drug users in Britain', in R. Battjes, and W. Pickens (eds) *Needle Sharing among Intravenous Drug Abusers: National and International Perspectives*, Washington: National Institute on Drug Abuse, Research Monograph Series 80.

Power, R., Hartnoll, R. and Daviaud, E. (1988) 'Drug injecting, AIDS, and risk behaviour: potential for change and intervention

strategies', *British Journal of Addiction* 83: 649–54.
Stall, R., McKusick, L. and Wiley, J. *et al.* (1986) 'Alcohol and drug use during sexual activity and compliance with safe sex guidelines for AIDS', *Health Education Quarterly* 13: 359–71.
Wijngaart, G. (1988) 'Heroin use in the Netherlands', *American Journal of Drug and Alcohol Abuse*, 14: 125–36.

Chapter Seven

CONTROL OF HIV INFECTION IN INJECTING DRUG USERS IN SAN FRANCISCO

ANDREW R. MOSS

The first clinical case of AIDS in an injecting drug user in San Francisco was diagnosed in 1983 and the number of cases diagnosed by the end of 1988 was 104. This compares with the 92 cases already diagnosed in homosexual men by the end of 1982, when AIDS studies began in San Francisco (Moss *et al.* 1983).

RECOGNITION OF THE DRUG USER EPIDEMIC

Until recently this drug user epidemic in San Francisco was dwarfed by the epidemic in homosexual men, and obscured by the fact that about 10 per cent of homosexual men with AIDS have injected drugs at least once. However, as the implications of HIV in drug users for the general heterosexual population have become clear, San Francisco has mounted a separate public health effort aimed at heterosexual injecting drug users. It would be misleading to describe this effort as a unified programme. In San Francisco, as in the United States in general, public health is a patchwork of separately funded state, local and federal interventions. What might best be described as a collage of programmes, organised by different entrepreneurs, was built up between 1984 and 1986, culminating in massive federal funding in 1986, when the catastrophic implications of the drug user epidemic had become apparent in Washington.

In late 1988 the Health Commissioner of New York City announced that the number of new AIDS cases in drug users had overtaken the number of new cases in homosexual men in that city. This phenomenon reflects the switch to safe sexual activity among gay men after the announcement of the AIDS epidemic in

1981. The flattening of AIDS incidence rates in gay men that followed some seven or eight years later is now visible in San Francisco, New York City and Los Angeles, the three main epidemic cities in the USA. As a result, AIDS in drug users has finally begun to overtake AIDS in gay men as the focus of public health in the American epidemic. In San Francisco, as in the rest of the USA and many European countries, the crossover in clinical case loads between gay men and drug users – which has many implications for the organisation of treatment – is likely to happen in the mid-1990s. In terms of prevention, however, drug users should already be the main target in many cities in America, Europe and elsewhere. New infections among San Francisco's 14,000 heterosexual injecting drug users are now some two or three times as frequent as they are among homosexual men.

STRATEGY

HIV testing and screening programme

Three separate programmes aimed at stopping the spread of HIV in drug users can be identified in San Francisco. The first was our systematic attempt in the AIDS Epidemiology Group at San Francisco General Hospital to screen injecting drug users in the city's methadone and detoxification programmes for HIV infection. This project, based on experience with the HIV antibody test in studies of homosexual men, was begun in 1985. It has screened 2,000 injecting drug users to date, and is now paralleled by a screening project in the 'street' setting organised by the Urban Health Study (Watters *et al.* 1988). Between the two groups 1,500 to 2,000 drug users are currently tested per year, being 10 to 15 per cent of the 'treatment population'. (The treatment population, the population of about 14,000 long-term heroin users who cycle through the treatment system, contains most AIDS cases in drug users and most known seropositives.)

We designed the HIV testing programme with two purposes in mind – both to collect data on HIV infection rates among users and also as an intervention. Seropositive drug users identified in the screening are recruited into follow-up where behavioural interventions can be brought to bear on them, their medical needs can be met, and their sexual partners can be recruited and screened.

About two-thirds of the drug users screened ask to be given their HIV results and about two-thirds of the positives so identified are recruited into follow-up. The increasing availability of treatment for people who are HIV seropositive will eventually increase these numbers.

This 'testing and follow-up' approach to prevention has taken several years to evolve even to its present somewhat fragmentary state. However, we are now on the threshold of delivering both primary medical care and sexually transmitted disease screening to injecting drug users and their sexual partners. All of the parts of this system, it should be noted, have to be funded separately.

Special treatment programmes for HIV-positive drug users

A second systematic intervention was based on the drug treatment programmes. In early 1986 the city of San Francisco funded treatment slots for HIV-positive drug users at several of the city's drug treatment programmes. A policy was adopted at the principal city methadone programme of giving priority to infected drug users. These decisions marked an important change of attitude among treatment providers, who had begun to realise that HIV in the addict population was the major problem facing them, rather than addiction itself. As with the HIV screening, the rationale for the slots is that the most effective targets for educational and behavioural intervention are the seropositive drug users and their sexual partners. One paradoxical result, however, is that it has become increasingly difficult for seronegative drug users to get into treatment.

Community health outreach worker programme

Finally, the third intervention in San Francisco, beginning in mid-1986, was the use of community health outreach workers to contact and give information to drug users on the street (Feldman and Biernacki 1988). The outreach programme provides a framework for other interventions such as a voucher system for immediate entry to drug treatment and an innovative attempt to distribute bleach to drug users for needle sterilisation. The bleach transaction provides a vehicle for discussion of safe needle use and other risk-minimisation behaviour. The project has as its symbolic centrepiece the figure of 'Bleachman', a costumed superhero who appears on the street distributing bleach.

ANALYSING THE HIV SEROPREVALENCE DATA

Demographic and drug use characteristics

Using the HIV seroprevalence and seroconversion data collected in the screenings, we have been able to establish the size and nature of the HIV-infected population (Chaisson *et al.* 1987; Moss and Chaisson 1988). We have also been able to collect data on effects of the interventions. In San Francisco as in other American cities the average age of the treatment population (HIV-seropositive as well as seronegative drug users) is 37, the median year of first heroin use is 1971, and the median number of times in treatment is five. The treatment population is thus a relatively middle-aged population of people who began using heroin in the late 1960s or early 1970s, are still using it intermittently, and cycle through the treatment programmes. Here the United States differs from many European countries, where most injecting drug users and also most HIV-seropositive drug users are in their twenties and began using heroin in the late 1970s or early 1980s. The implications from the screening data for intervention are manifold; for example, it is highly unlikely that middle-aged drug users with 15 to 20 years in and out of treatment are going to respond in large numbers to interventions based on abstinence.

Extent and timing of HIV infection

Alarmingly many of the HIV-seropositive drug users we have identified are relatively far advanced in the course of the disease. Twelve of the first 100 seropositives identified had a CD4 lymphocytes count of less than 200 and thus were eligible for zidovudine (AZT) therapy under current guidelines; only one is known to have received it. HIV-infected drug users are one of the most medically underserved populations in the United States.

About 15 per cent of drug users in San Francisco are now seropositive – that would be about 2,000 HIV-positive drug users in the city. We have found very little evidence of infection in young people: of 250 seropositive drug users identified to date, only ten were under 25 years old. Seropositive drug users are more likely to be black or Hispanic than drug users in general, and are far more likely to inject cocaine. In a recent study we found that many heroin users in methadone treatment were using cocaine, that about a quarter had begun using cocaine since entry to methadone treatment, and that intravenous cocaine use was the most powerful predictor of HIV seropositivity (Chaisson *et al.* 1989). These findings reflect the movement of cocaine from the middle class to the urban poor in the United States. The association of HIV seropositivity and cocaine use is particularly worrying because some fraction of the current generation of young 'crack' users will probably graduate to inject cocaine. Currently the greatest natural boundary to the future spread of HIV in the United States is sexual segregation by age. HIV-infected crack users would provide a route for the virus to move from the largely middle-aged population which is infected now to the younger, sexually active crack users who are currently uninfected.

THE SAN FRANCISCO HIV SEROCONVERSION STUDY

The screening studies have become increasingly unrepresentative as the drug user population has adapted to our testing and to the virus. Among men at least, many of the HIV seropositives have by now either been found by us and diverted, or decided not to be tested (all testing is voluntary and anonymous). Thus, the observed seropositivity rate has begun to decline. Such an apparent decline is common when a population is studied repeatedly, and has been observed in the US military induction and blood bank studies. It does not reflect a real decline in infection. We therefore began a seroconversion study to keep track of new infection in the drug user population.

Although the HIV testing programme is anonymous, unique identifiers are taken, and HIV seroconversion rates can be calculated among subjects who happen to have been studied twice or more. Figure 7.1 gives preliminary seroconversion rates over time in 220 such subjects studied twice during 1985–8. Based on these rather scanty data, it appears that the estimated annual seroconversion rate fell during 1985–6, but remained stable at about 3 per cent per year in 1987–8, leading to estimates of about 350 new infections per year among the 12,000 uninfected drug users in the treatment population in the last two years. (This number can be compared with an estimated 0.5 per cent seroconversion rate per year in 20,000 uninfected homosexual men, or about 100 new infections a year in 1988.)

Figure 7.1 Estimated HIV seroconversion rates among San Francisco drug users in treatment

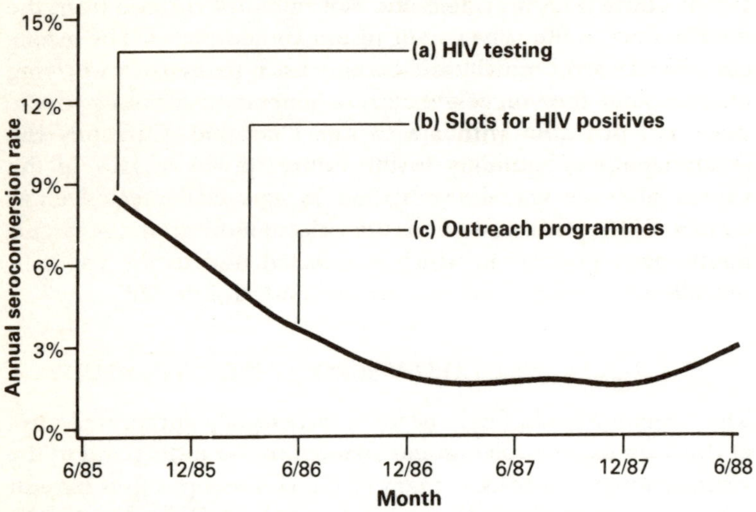

Notes:
(a) Date of commencement of HIV screening in drug treatment programmes.
(b) Date of opening of treatment programme slots for HIV seropositives.
(c) Date of beginnng of community health worker outreach programmes.

Points (a), (b) and (c) in Figure 7.1 show the start dates of the three main interventions described above. Although the data in this figure are preliminary, they suggest that the seroconversion rate was heading downward in 1985, probably as a result of media attention to the epidemic, and that the effect of this attention together with the three interventions was to produce the current rate of 3 per cent per year. Much of the reduction was clearly attributable to the publicising of the epidemic alone.

Data associated with the bleach distribution programme

Specific information is available on the bleach distribution programme. About 80 per cent of the drug users in the drug treatment programmes admitted sharing needles in 1988, and about half of those who admit such sharing now claim to use bleach 'regularly' or 'always' to clean their equipment. However, HIV seropositivity rates were comparable in those who did and those who did not use bleach (Table 7.1), so that as yet the bleach programme has not shown itself to have had any effect on HIV seropositivity. This may be a result of the relative newness of the programme, and the fact that drug users have been seroconverting for HIV since at least 1977. Some very recent data are more encouraging; they suggest that using bleach for more than two years is associated with a very low seropositivity rate. Less encouraging is fragmentary evidence that HIV seropositivity (in women drug users at least) is associated with sexual-exposure risk factors. HIV may now be recognisably a sexually transmitted disease amongst injecting drug users.

Table 7.1 HIV seropositivity rate by bleach use among injecting drug users who admitted ever sharing needles (1986–8)

	HIV seropositivity rate (%) among subjects who used bleach	
	Never or rarely	*Sometimes or always*
1988	8	11
1987	14	12
1986	10	10

CONCLUSION

The San Francisco HIV seroconversion data are encouraging since they suggest that new infections can be brought to a low level by relatively easy interventions like those described above. There seems to be no doubt that a high proportion of injecting drug users in the treatment programme population can change their drug use so as to reduce markedly their risk of HIV infection. Probably interventions other than those used in San Francisco would produce comparable rates – e.g. needle exchanges where they are politically acceptable, or mass advertising campaigns, as in the UK.

However, a more intensive approach may be needed with those drug users who are not responding to the current approaches.

Probably we should be seeking out HIV-seropositive drug users and other people at high risk, rather than waiting for them to come to us through the drug treatment system. In San Francisco the politics of HIV testing in homosexual men has changed gradually over the past five years, reflecting the fact that many HIV-positive individuals are reaching the stage of developing clinical disease, and also reflecting the fact that AZT and aerosolised-pentamidine have become available as out-patient therapies. Most physicians in San Francisco are now encouraging their gay patients to be tested. Many infected injecting drug users are now increas- ingly likely to develop clinical disease. Since this population is badly underserved, political hesitations about seeking out HIV seropositives are probably already barring at least some eligible persons from treatment. The balance between the benefit of deliverable therapy and the fear of being found to be HIV seropositive is shifting gradually for those who are infected with HIV. As the balance shifts, the public health approach to HIV infection in drug users should probably shift too, tilting gradually away from broad educational interventions and towards a more traditional sexually transmitted disease approach to prevention – the approach of going out to find and treat infected drug users and their sexual partners.

REFERENCES

Chaisson, R.E., Bacchetti, P., Osmond, D., Brodie, B., Sande, M.A. and Moss, A.R. (1989) 'Cocaine use and HIV infection in intravenous drug users in San Francisco', *Journal of the American Medical Association* 261: 561–5.

Chaisson, R., Moss, A.R., Onishi, R. *et al.* (1987) 'Human Immunodeficiency Virus infection in heterosexual intravenous drug users in San Francisco', *American Journal of Public Health* 77: 169–72.

Feldman, H.W. and Biernacki, P. (1988) 'The ethnography of needle sharing among intravenous drug users and implications for public policies and intervention strategies', in R. Battjes, and R.W. Pickens (eds) *Needle Sharing among Intravenous Drug Users, National and International Perspectives*, Washington: National Institute on Drug Abuse, Research Monograph Series 80.

Moss, A.R., Bacchetti, P., Gorman, M., Dritz, S., Conant, C., Abrams, D. *et al.* (1983) 'AIDS in the "gay" areas of San Francisco', *Lancet* i: 923–4.

Moss, A.R. and Chaisson, R.E. (1988) 'AIDS and intravenous drug use in San Francisco', in D. Des Jarlais (ed.) *AIDS and Public Policy* 3 (3).
Watters, J.K., Case, P., Huang, K., Cheng, Y-T., Lorvick, J. and Carlson, J. (1988) 'HIV Seroepidemiology and Behaviour Change in Intravenous Drug Users: Progress Report on the Effectiveness of Street-based Prevention', Stockholm: Fourth International Conference on AIDS, Abstract 8523.

Chapter Eight

THE EPIDEMIC OF HIV INFECTION AMONG INJECTING DRUG USERS IN NEW YORK CITY: THE FIRST DECADE AND POSSIBLE FUTURE DIRECTIONS

DON C. DES JARLAIS AND SAMUEL R. FRIEDMAN

The epidemic of HIV-1 among intravenous drug users in New York City has been of particular public health importance for several reasons. First, there is the sheer size of this epidemic. Our best current estimates indicate that there are approximately 100,000 injecting drug users who have already been exposed to the virus, and there are an estimated 100,000 more at high risk of becoming exposed. Second, there is the length of time that the virus has been present among injecting drug users in the city – over a decade. Compared to other cities, the history of the HIV epidemic among injecting drug users in New York is thus very advanced, and there are undoubtedly many ways in which the New York epidemic may be repeated (albeit sometimes on a smaller scale) in other locations. In this chapter, we will trace the history of the epidemic, and note current trends with an eye to the future of the epidemic. (The historical section is adapted from Des Jarlais *et al.* in press).

HISTORY OF HIV TRANSMISSION AMONG INJECTING DRUG USERS IN NEW YORK CITY

Figure 8.1 shows our historical reconstruction of the spread of HIV-1 among injecting drug users from 1975 through 1987. This reconstruction is based on the early cases of AIDS reported to the New York City Department of Health and our seroprevalence surveys. The points on the figure represent actual data from the seroprevalence surveys, while the bars are interpolated seroprevalence rates using the AIDS case data and the trend since

Figure 8.1 Historical reconstruction of HIV-I seroprevalence among active injecting drug users in Manhattan, New York City*

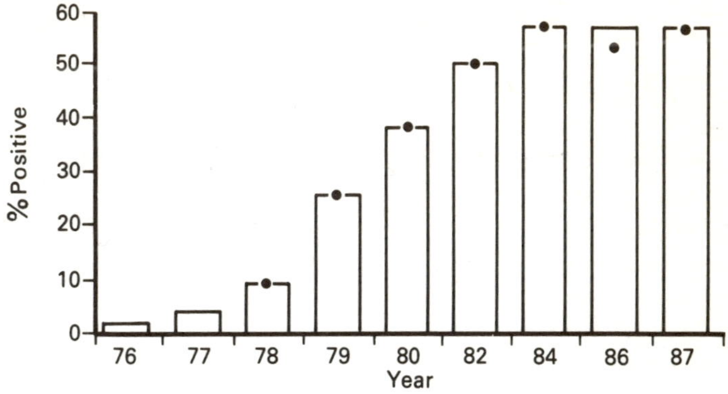

Source: Adapted from Des Jarlais *et al.* in press

Note: *Bars represent historical reconstruction. Points reflect data from surveys of injecting drug users entering treatment programmes.

1984. The spread of HIV-1 has been represented by a sigmoid curve typical of the diffusion of infectious diseases through populations.

The first 'hard' evidence for HIV-1 infection among injecting drug users in New York is from three cases of paediatric AIDS in children born in 1977. These cases were later reported to the New York City Department of Health AIDS surveillance unit. These children were born to mothers known to be injecting drug users, and the children had no other known risks for AIDS.

The earliest known case of AIDS in an adult injecting drug user occurred in 1979, in a male who also had homosexual activity as a risk behaviour. The first five known cases among heterosexual injecting drug users occurred in 1980, when there were an additional three cases with both injecting drug use and male homosexual activity as risk behaviours. Cases among injecting drug users increased rapidly from the eight in 1980, to 31 in 1981, to 160 in 1982, and to 340 in 1983.

It appears that the HIV-1 epidemic among injecting drug users in New York City can be divided into three phases: an introduction/initial spread phase, followed by a phase of rapid spread, followed by the current relative stabilisation phase. The three cases in 1977 of apparent perinatal transmission from injecting drug-using women strongly suggest that the introduction of HIV-1 into the injecting drug user group occurred around 1975 or 1976, or perhaps even earlier.

HIV-1 was probably introduced into the injecting drug use group in New York from homosexual/bisexual men, with homosexual/bisexual injecting drug users serving as a bridge group. The earliest known adult cases of AIDS were all among homosexual/bisexual men not known to have injected drugs, and a very high percentage of homosexual/bisexual men were among the first known cases among injecting drug users. If male homosexual/bisexual injecting drug users did serve as a bridge from homosexual/bisexual men who did not inject drugs to heterosexual injecting drug users, it is likely that there were multiple points of introduction of HIV-1 into the heterosexual injecting drug use group in New York.

During this initial phase of the HIV-1 epidemic among injecting drug users in New York, there undoubtedly was a spread of HIV-1, but most sharing of drug injection equipment was probably among persons who had not been exposed to the virus. There are no extensive serum samples from this period, and so it is not possible to be certain about the spread of HIV-1 among injecting drug users, but our later studies suggest that the seroprevalence rate remained below 20 per cent for the first three to four years after the introduction of the virus into the injecting drug user group in the city.

Based on the seroprevalence data from the samples collected from 1978 through 1983, and the rapid rise in clinical cases from 1980 through 1983, a second phase occurred from approximately 1978 through 1981. This phase was characterised by a rapid rise in the seroprevalence rate, from less than 20 per cent prior to this phase to about 50 per cent at the end of the period. Similar periods of rapid spread of HIV-1 among injecting drug users have been reported from elsewhere (see Chapters 9 and 10). In New York, several factors may have contributed to this rapid spread during this time. In the late 1970s and early 1980s there was a substantial increase in the supply of both heroin and cocaine in the New York area. This led to increases in the injection of both drugs, primarily among persons who already had histories of injecting heroin. Frequency of injection of these drugs has been linked to seropositivity among injecting drug users in Manhattan (Marmor *et al.*

1987). Manhattan also has numerous 'shooting galleries', places where one may rent drug injection equipment, use it, and then return it to the gallery owner for rental to the next customer. The use of shooting galleries provides a mechanism for the spread of HIV to large numbers of other injecting drug users and also has been linked to HIV exposure (Marmor *et al.* 1987).

Since 1983, the HIV-1 epidemic among injecting drug users in Manhattan appears to have entered a phase with relatively stable seroprevalence rates among injecting drug users entering treatment. There has been no increase observed in the seroprevalence rates from 1984 through 1987. This relative stabilisation of the HIV-1 seroprevalence rate among injecting drug users entering treatment in Manhattan does not mean that there are no new HIV infections among injecting drug users in the area. New HIV-1 exposures are also occurring among current injecting drug users in New York City. Our own cohort study shows an annual rate of new infections of approximately 5 per cent among subjects who were initially seronegative (Des Jarlais *et al.* 1987) and an ongoing cohort study in the Bronx has found a similar seroconversion rate.

This stabilisation of the HIV-1 seroprevalence rate, while not implying an absence of new infections, is at a level that is much below what would be expected from hepatitis B exposure rates. Seroprevalence rates for hepatitis B range from 80 per cent to 95 per cent among injecting drug users in New York. The lower seroprevalence rate for HIV-1 compared to hepatitis B is consistent with hepatitis B virus being easier to transmit through microtransfusions (Gerberding *et al.* 1985). The current seroprevalence rate for HIV-1 is also much below what would be expected from basic models of diffusion of infectious agents. Under the assumption of random mixing of infected and non-infected persons in these models, the increase in seroprevalence is highest when half of the population is infected and half is not infected (Bailey 1975).

ENTERING A PERIOD OF STABILISATION

The current relative stabilisation of HIV seroprevalence among injecting drug users in New York is clearly a complex resultant of multiple factors. From our analyses, there are at least three factors that have created the relative stabilisation.

One factor is the *loss of HIV-seropositive drug users from the pool of active injecting drug users.* Loss of seropositives would both reduce the spread of the virus to uninfected injecting drug users, and, of course, reduce the absolute number of seropositives likely to be found in any sample of recent or current injecting drug users. Seropositive drug users may stop injecting through a variety of mechanisms, including successful drug abuse treatment, stopping injection through their own efforts, and development of disease and death. From our ongoing cohort study, we would estimate that approximately 3 per cent of seropositives per year are lost from active injecting drug use through the development of AIDS and other fatal illnesses (Des Jarlais *et al.* 1987).

A second factor would be *conscious AIDS risk reductions.* AIDS-related behaviour change is believed to be the primary cause of stabilisation of HIV-1 seroprevalence rates among homosexual/bisexual men in San Francisco (see Chapter 7) and risk reduction is likely to be playing a part in the observed stability of HIV-1 seroprevalence among injecting drug users in Manhattan. Several studies have shown AIDS risk reduction among injecting drug users in New York City (Des Jarlais *et al.* 1985; Friedman *et al.* 1987; Selwyn *et al.* 1987). There is also evidence of increasing behaviour change among injecting drug users in Manhattan over the period in which the seroprevalence rates have remained at their current level. In 1984, 59 per cent of the methadone patients in a study by Friedman *et al.* (1987) stated that they had made some form of behaviour change in order to reduce the risk of AIDS. When the same question was asked in 1986 of patients who had recently entered methadone maintenance treatment, 75 per cent stated that they had changed their behaviour, and when the question was asked of patients entering an experimental methadone programme in 1987, 85 per cent replied that they had changed their behaviour (Des Jarlais *et al.* in press).

The final factor that is probably contributing to the observed stability of seroprevalence rates among injecting drug users in Manhattan is the *entry of new injecting drug users into the group.* Persons who begin injecting drugs are very unlikely to be HIV-1 seropositive before they begin; continued entry of new users into the injecting drug use group would therefore help stabilise the seroprevalence rate below 100 per cent saturation. Our best estimates are that enough enter to replace those leaving, approximately 5 per cent to 10 per cent per year.

MONITORING FUTURE TRENDS IN SEROPREVALENCE

There are several trends regarding seroprevalence/risk behaviours that need to be monitored in New York.

While the HIV seroprevalence has remained relatively stable among injecting drug users over the last four years, the epidemic should not be considered 'over'. There are several recent developments that could transform the epidemic of HIV among drug users in New York. These developments will require careful monitoring in the short- and intermediate-term future.

There is an increasing association of cocaine injection and HIV exposure. In a recent study of seroconversions in our cohort, cocaine injection was significantly related to becoming seropositive, while heroin injection was not (Des Jarlais and Friedman 1988); cocaine injection was also associated with higher initial HIV seroprevalence rates than was heroin injection in a recent study of one of our AIDS outreach prevention projects in New York.

Possible historical changes in the associations between specific injected drugs and HIV are suggested by the fact that cocaine injection was not an independent predictor of HIV exposure in our 1984 data (Marmor *et al.* 1987).

Cocaine may play a particularly important role in spreading HIV. Its pattern of injection (often at very high frequencies, approximately every ten minutes, until the supply is exhausted) makes decontamination of shared injection equipment very difficult, increasing the potential for HIV transmission.

Since there is no modality that utilises a pharmacological cross-tolerance 'blockade' for cocaine, treatment for cocaine dependence is particularly difficult.

In addition to the cocaine linkage to HIV transmission, there are potential difficulties in maintaining risk reduction. Our studies have shown that a steadily increasing percentage of injecting drug users in New York have changed their behaviour in order to reduce their risks of developing AIDS. The extent to which this AIDS risk reduction can be consolidated and maintained indefinitely is an open empirical question. Certainly the drug abuse treatment literature shows that maintaining behaviour change among injecting drug users is much more difficult than making the initial change.

In one of our current studies, 25 per cent of subjects recruited from a southern Manhattan street setting reported that they had not been able to maintain their initial form of AIDS risk reduction. Preliminary analyses of these data suggest that failure to maintain risk reduction is associated with a denial of the likelihood of being exposed to HIV.

Because large numbers of injecting drug users in New York have already been exposed to HIV, there will undoubtedly be increasing numbers of injecting drug users who will develop full-blown AIDS over the next several years. How this increased number of cases will affect AIDS risk reduction is an important question. Studies of gay men suggest that the presence of large numbers of cases within the community fosters risk reduction but also that this situation creates intense psychological stress within members of the group. For injecting drug users, particularly those not in treatment programmes, intense stress might lead to increased drug use, a traditional method of coping with stress.

The ability of injecting drug users to maintain AIDS risk reduction over long periods, particularly as the number of cases increases, will be important for planning AIDS prevention efforts in all cities that already have or do develop high seroprevalence rates among their injecting drug users. The epidemic among injecting drug users in New York is continuing through heterosexual transmission from injecting drug users. While injecting drug users have been fairly quick to change injection behaviour to reduce the risk of developing AIDS, they have been very slow to change their heterosexual behaviour. At present there are insufficient data for selecting among several potential explanations for this slowness in changing heterosexual behaviour (see review in Des Jarlais and Friedman in press).

In our New York studies, we have seen small but steady increases in the percentage of injecting drug users who have changed their heterosexual behaviour because of concerns about AIDS – from 14 per cent in 1984 to approximately 40 per cent in 1987–8. From our current analyses, peer support appears to be a very important factor in changing heterosexual behaviour of injecting drug users. Important questions will include specifying under what conditions this peer support influences risk reduction, determining whether the trend will continue over a longer time period, and more generally understanding the determinants of and obstacles to heterosexual behaviour change.

A final concern regards changes in transmissibility. There is preliminary evidence that the infectiousness of seropositive persons increases as they move towards developing full-blown AIDS. If this occurs on a large scale, then one would expect later waves of transmission as more seropositive injecting drug users in New York become more infectious as they begin to become clinically ill.

CONCLUSION

The epidemic of HIV among injecting drug users in New York City has already gone through three distinguishable phases. The introductory stage was followed by a stage of rapid spread which was followed by a stage of relative stabilisation in seroprevalence. Each of these stages has lasted from three to five years. This current stage of relative stabilisation may or may not continue.

A number of emerging factors, from injection of cocaine through increased infectiousness, could radically change the present situation of relative stability in HIV seroprevalence among injecting drug users in New York. The factors cited are not meant to be a comprehensive listing of potentially important factors for the future of HIV transmission among and from injecting drug users in New York, but are meant to illustrate various possibilities for the future of the HIV epidemic among injecting drug users in the city. Despite the high and currently stable rate of HIV seroprevalence among injecting drug users in New York, the epidemic is not 'over'. Continued monitoring of the HIV epidemic among injecting drug users in New York is important because of the sheer size of the problem within the city and the possibility for using knowledge obtained from New York to develop effective AIDS prevention programming elsewhere.

REFERENCES

Bailey, N.T.J. (1975) *The Mathematical Theory of Infectious Diseases and its Applications*, New York: Hafner Press.

Des Jarlais, D.C. and Friedman, S.R. (1988) 'HIV infection among persons who inject illicit drugs: problems and prospects', *Journal of the Acquired Immune Deficiency Syndrome*, 1: 267–73.

Des Jarlais, D.C. and Friedman, S.R. (in press) 'AIDS 88: HIV and intravenous drug use', *AIDS*.

Des Jarlais, D.C., Friedman, S.R. and Hopkins, W. (1985) 'Risk reduction for the Acquired Immunodeficiency Syndrome among intravenous drug users', *Annals of Internal Medicine* 103: 755–9.

Des Jarlais, D.C., Friedman, S.R., Marmor, M., Cohen, H., Mildvan, D., Yancovitz, S., Mathur, U., El-Sadr, W., Spira, T.J., Garber, J., Beatrice, S.T., Abdul-Quader, A.S. and Sotheran, J.L. (1987) 'Development of AIDS, HIV seroconversion, and co-factors for T4 cell loss in a cohort of intravenous drug users', *AIDS* 1: 105–11.

Des Jarlais, D.C., Friedman, S.R., Novick, D., Sotheran, J.L., Yancovitz, S.R., Mildvan, D., Weber, J., Kreek, M.J., Maslansky, R., Spira, T., Thomas, P. and Marmor, M. (in press) 'HIV-1 infection among intravenous drug users in Manhattan', *Journal of the American Medical Association*.

Friedman, S.R., Des Jarlais, D.C., Sotheran, J.L., Garber, J., Cohen, H. and Smith, D. (1987) 'AIDS and self-organization among intravenous drug users', *International Journal of the Addictions* 22: 201–20.

Gerberding, J.L., Hopewell, P.C., Kaminsky, L.S. and Sande, M.A. (1985) 'Transmission of Hepatitis B without transmission of AIDS by accidental needlestick', *New England Journal of Medicine*, 312: 56.

Marmor, M., Des Jarlais, D.C., Cohen, H., Friedman, S.R., Beatrice, S.T., Dubin, N., El-Sadr, W., Mildvan, D., Yancovitz, S., Mathur, U. and Holzman, R. (1987) 'Risk factors for infection with Human Immunodeficiency Virus among intravenous drug abusers in New York City', *AIDS* 1: 39–44.

Selwyn, P.A., Feiner, C., Cox, C.P., Lipschutz, C. and Cohen, R. (1987) 'Knowledge about AIDS and high-risk behavior among intravenous drug abusers in New York City', *AIDS* 1: 247–54.

Chapter Nine

THE EDINBURGH EPIDEMIC: A CASE STUDY

ROY ROBERTSON

Understanding the events giving rise to the current situation of AIDS in drug users in Edinburgh requires a historic perspective. Drug injecting was present in this region prior to the arrival of HIV, as it was in many other UK and international centres, and pre-AIDS research had identified problem drug takers in both east and west Scotland (Ditton and Speirits 1982; Ward 1971; Woodside 1973). What was perhaps different was the rapid increase in the number of drug injectors over a short period of time immediately prior to the introduction of HIV and the comparative lack of appropriate services set up to respond to this injecting drug use. The consequence of this combination of events was a large number of extremely inexperienced drug users with a readily accessible supply of good-quality heroin, out of touch with agencies likely to influence behaviour for the better or able to provide equipment to enable non-septic techniques to prevail.

LITTLE PROBLEM; LITTLE SERVICE

Historically, services had been provided for drug users at the local psychiatric hospital which is the designated drug treatment centre for Lothian region. On the plus side, the presence of a single centre of secondary referral and little active treatment facilities made the drug problem more easily visible in its entirety (Woodside 1973). Originally, back in the late 1960s, consultants were identified and licensed to prescribe heroin for addicts and over the early years a range of approaches were tried, including withdrawal programmes using intravenous and oral drugs, in-patient reduction under supervision and psychiatric support as out-patients. On the minus side, in the late 1970s and early 1980s people working in this service became disillusioned and disappointed with results and felt that the 1982 report on *Treatment and Rehabilitation* from the Advisory Council on the Misuse of Drugs (ACMD) confirmed the correctness of their decision to move away from a formal psychiatric medical model of treatment to a multidisciplinary, community-based approach. During 1983 and 1984 the establishment of a Joint Working Party on Drug Abuse allowed for the delay in establishment of alternative services which in retrospect left the responsibility for any decisive action vacant. The subsequent report *Drugs Action Lothian* which appeared in March 1986 was already superseded by the awareness of the HIV problems and by the extensive recommendations to establish the range of educational, medical, social work and community facilities along the lines laid out in the two ACMD reports (1982 and 1984). This complicated evolutionary change in service provision, combined with bureaucratic delay, left a hiatus in service provision during a critical time in history. A window of opportunity for the Human Immunodeficiency Virus was opened and, in common with other infectious diseases, the advantage was taken and spread was rapid.

THE GROWTH OF A 'DRUG PROBLEM'

Throughout the 1980s, a study has been carried out in a community setting to observe the wider spectrum of drug problems in a distinct catchment area rather than just those problems requiring specialist advice. The problems presenting to a general practice through a decade of observation ranged from the problematic stereotype drug addict, seen so often in drug dependence units, to the individuals who had tried drugs for a short period only, the ephemeral drug user and the relatives and friends with concerns and problems secondary to drug abuse. A perspective not usually recorded was that of the families, children and community reaction to a wave of drug misuse.

During the 1970s, drug misuse in Edinburgh had developed gradually from a culture using pharmaceutically prepared drugs obtained from retail or wholesale supplies to an increasingly injection-orientated problem. Anecdotal evidence from doctors, law enforcement agencies and drug users suggests that, throughout the 1970s, numbers of individuals injecting drugs rose from 50 or so to several hundred by 1979. Drugs being injected included amphetamine, barbiturates, diconal (dipipanone/cyclizine combination) and heroin. The supply largely depended on London contacts rather than the independently emerging drug scene in the west of Scotland. The problems therefore reflected those in the south and probably existed as a subsidiary of the larger London centre. Supplies were available in city centre pubs and a small number of private houses, but had not yet moved to the large sprawling council housing schemes on the periphery of the city.

The later change in distribution pattern was important to subsequent events. Changing events after this time were by no means unique to Edinburgh. Glasgow experienced a rapid increase in drug injecting in the early 1980s (Ditton and Speirits 1982) as did Dundee and many English towns. Across Europe, it is now known, many countries became aware of new problems related to drug injecting.

International developments appeared to make heroin readily available throughout Europe and the presence of such a commodity, associated with a profound ignorance of the effects and dangers, allowed consumer demand to expand rapidly. In 1982 many 17- or 18-year-old adolescents were heard to remark that they knew more contemporaries who injected drugs than did not, and could obtain heroin at many places within a short distance from their homes in Edinburgh. Drugs were sold cheaply and initially unhindered by effective police activity; treatment centres were unprepared and overwhelmed by the sudden demand for support by families and relatives. Experiencing little problems in the 'honeymoon period' of heroin use, the majority of drug takers felt little need for help or support.

STAMPING OUT NEEDLE AND SYRINGE AVAILABILITY

During the early 1980s there was negligible understanding by drug users of the problems associated with injecting and sharing. This was exemplified by the willingness of those individuals to rent or borrow bloodstained needles and syringes, inject fluid contaminated with blood and to use glass pipettes and other makeshift injecting apparatus to administer intravenous injections. Prior to 1982 several sources of clean injecting equipment existed, but as demand and associated problems escalated, and in line with restrictive recommendations from the Pharmaceutical Association, supplies dwindled at a critical time. The last surviving enthusiastic retail supplier was forced out of business in late 1982 (Henderson 1985) and the self-reported incidence of dangerous needle sharing escalated further. In his final year of business this pharmaceutical supplier reports selling needles and syringes to a large number of individuals who he knew injected; at times he sold boxes of 100 to people who supplied the market. Although this problem clearly was critical to subsequent events the lack of interest in clean equipment demonstrated by drug users throughout the ensuing wave of hepatitis B was frustrating to many health professionals. Through this time police activity included an informal policy of trying to cut out the availability of any needles and syringes and in this way reduce the extent of injectible drug use. Although well intentioned, this practice may have encouraged sharing of injecting equipment to become the norm amongst drug users, for all but one out of 200 addicts interviewed in the mid-1980s were taking their drugs by injecting – a popularity of injecting far higher than in most parts of the UK.

THE ARRIVAL AND RAPID SPREAD OF HIV

The single feature which distinguishes the Edinburgh situation from other centres in the UK is the speed with which transmission occurred in the group of known drug users (Figure 9.1). Although it is assumed that spread was predominantly by sharing of contaminated needles and syringes, there was undoubtedly a similarly rapid transmission of virus heterosexually occurring within this group but also involving non-drug users.

Thus, two epidemics occurring at the same time in a large group of young people were subsequently charted by testing of stored samples of blood largely taken for hepatitis B testing. Many case records from that period noted glandular-fever-like illnesses but failed to find the classical marker of the Epstein-Barr virus (the illness we know now was an HIV seroconversion illness). Later testing has identified a further number of HIV-antibody-positive individuals, but many presenting with positive tests are known to have used drugs since 1983 and therefore may have been infected at any time subsequent to then. The timing of the epidemic of HIV infection in this group was between late 1983 and 1985 (see

Figure 9.1 Cumulative number of first positive HIV antibody results amongst 83 injecting drug users

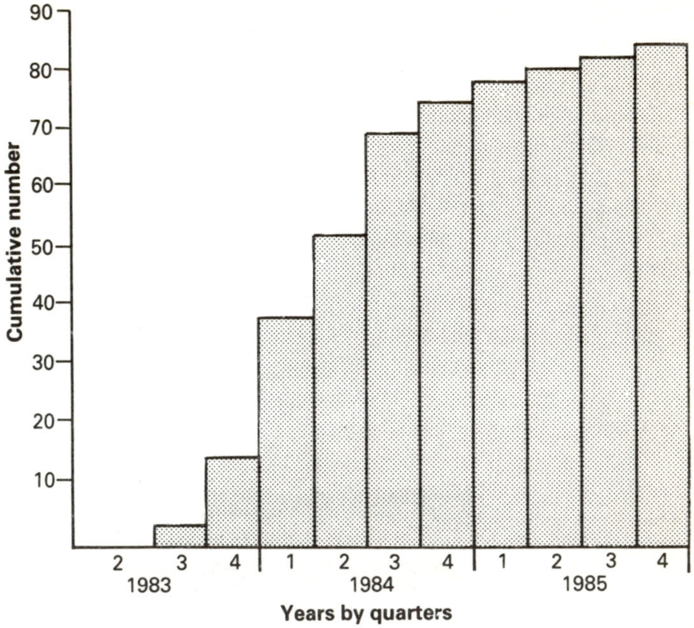

Figures 9.1 and 9.2). Figure 9.2 illustrates those positive by year of starting to inject drugs. Both these figures suggest that most of those currently known to be HIV positive became so during this period. Also, although seroconversions continue to be observed, these are in keeping with an endemic pattern of spread rather than an epidemic. Most recently recorded seroconversions have been attributed to heterosexual transmission rather than drug use. It may be that history will record a heterosexual epidemic occurring subsequent to the drug-associated epidemic of HIV.

If not abundantly clear now, the lesson from these findings will become so during the next few years as symptomatic cases arise. At the present time such clinical problems are among non-drug users, children and long-term abstainers from drug use as well as those actively addicted. Interestingly, the management problems for Edinburgh are still being explored in terms of prevention as many drug users have changed their behaviour and are now less at risk from drug-using behaviour than from their sexual behaviour.

Figure 9.2 Injecting drug users found to be HIV-positive according to the year of first injecting

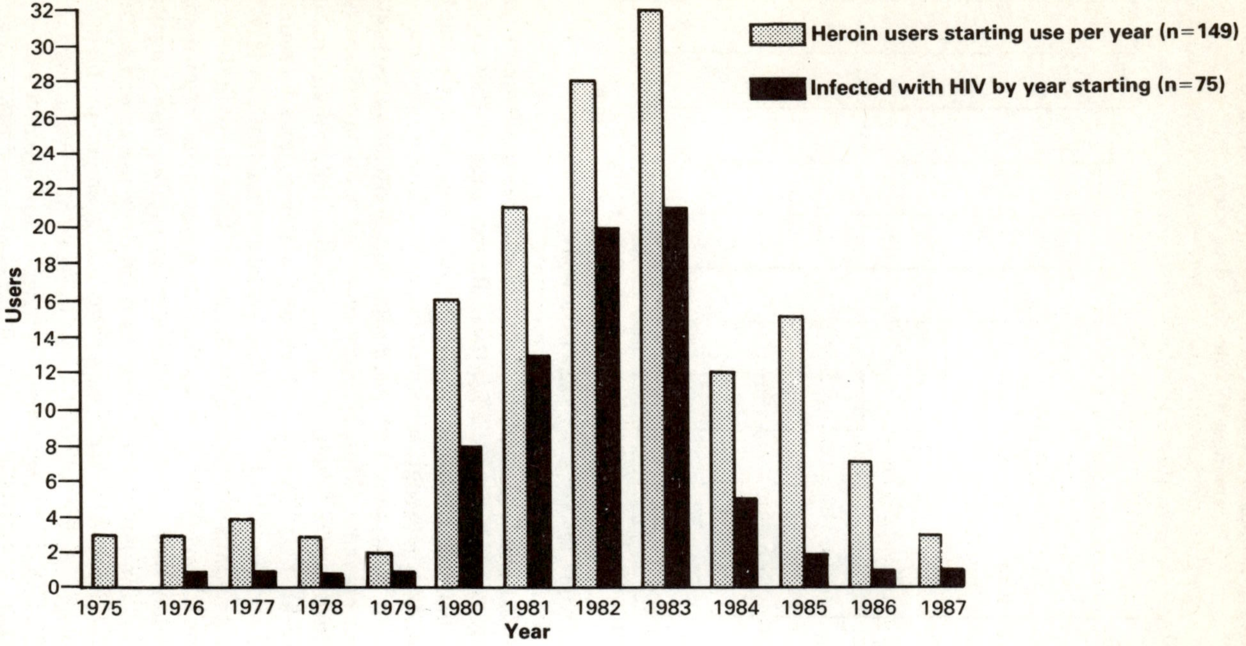

PROFESSIONALS' VIEWS ON DRUG PROBLEMS

When trying to understand the attitudes today compared with those prevalent in the early 1980s, it is interesting to remember that prior to AIDS the drug debate centred very much on the importance of controlling drug misuse by legal constraint versus the possibility of control by appropriate treatment and education (Stimson and Oppenheimer 1982). This diversity of approach is illustrated by two quotations at that time. The Solicitor General for Scotland stated that:

> The hope is that, firstly, we will get closer to the end of the chain [of supply] and secondly that it will begin to get across that it is hopeless, that you can't claim that you were just a small fry in the organisation and you are still going to be prosecuted in the High Court . . . I welcome the idea of moving the minimum sentence up from 14 years to life.
>
> (*Glasgow Herald*, 19 February 1985)

In contrast, a leading defence lawyer in Edinburgh (who represented many drug users charged with drug dealing despite having been in possession of as little as 1–2 grams of heroin) explained:

> These people [in court] are invariably heroin addicts whose habit has forced them into crime and connection with bigger fish . . . The Government should be spending the money that is being spent on keeping people in prison in the community. I think it now costs £150–£200 per day to keep someone in prison.
>
> (*Glasgow Herald*, 19 February 1985)

The first statement clearly reflected the prevailing political line (spelt out in more detail in *Tackling Drug Misuse*, a document published by the Home Office in 1985). This concentrated hard on control and had little to say or recommend to comfort the individual with an addiction problem.

This debate, in which many professionals participated, was largely about a non-medical approach to a problem which was seen as a problem of control and public order. Attempts therefore to provide sterile equipment or to present policies based on damage limitation were at the time regarded as, at best, eccentric or by others as problematic. Under a typically hysterical headline of

'War we must win' the following quotation appeared in a national daily newspaper:

> It is a crazy world where, 24 hours after a young man is found dead in his home from an overdose of heroin, a doctor admits he gives syringes to patients in the knowledge that they use them to inject drugs. Why?
> "Because it is better than them running the risk of catching Hepatitis" he argues.
> What bilge!
> It is this confused thinking which undermines all efforts to fight the war against drugs, ruthlessly and relentlessly.
> (*Daily Express*, 26 April 1985)

The attention of the public and the medical profession was drawn very much therefore to the need for legal, political and social control and consequently diverted from the outstanding need for medical assessment, detoxification and treatment facilities, education and compassionate care of all involved. These considerations were seen at the time as wasteful, unnecessary and even counterproductive.

Nowhere in the UK was this non-medical attitude towards drug misuse and drug abusers more intensely felt than in Scotland. In the absence of a single psychiatrist actively involved in treatment, Edinburgh and Dundee were most severely affected. Indeed, the situation was so disturbing that an entire chapter was devoted to the Scottish situation in the 1988 report on *AIDS and Drug Misuse* from the UK's Advisory Council on the Misuse of Drugs.

THE ORIGINS OF THE EPIDEMIC

The putative cause of the Edinburgh epidemic of HIV transmission in injecting drug users must be this combination of events: a large immature drug-injecting subculture with little experience of illegal substances, together with a comparative absence of services which might influence behaviour. In addition, an extremely active law enforcement initiative designed to suppress and control the problem gave rise to a scarcity of needles and syringes. The increasing legal constraints on those found guilty of drug- related crimes allowed for an increasing number of prison sentences, during which time drugs were often injected in an even more damaging series of circumstances (see Chapter 18). Anecdotes persist of extensive drug injecting in many Scottish prisons in which languished a staggering number of known drug users. Into this environment at its peak came the Human Immunodeficiency Virus.

Although there were occasional expressions of anxiety, the medical establishment was to remain in ignorance of this epidemic until late 1985, when antibody testing for HIV became available. As in other centres and risk groups, the factor that facilitated the extensive and invisible epidemic was the long asymptomatic period associated with HIV and AIDS. Indeed, without the ability to detect antibody very few cases would have been detected before 1987. Even at the time of writing, the majority of infected drug users, children and sexual partners remain in the asymptomatic or early symptomatic phase of infection. The number of deaths attributable to AIDS is still greatly outnumbered by the traditional fatal problems of drug injecting – namely, suicide, violence and accidental overdose. This balance is likely to change profoundly towards a large number of HIV-related deaths from now on and for the foreseeable future.

CHANGES IN THE DRUG OF USE

During the early 1980s another pattern has unfolded among local drug users. This is a progression of drugs of abuse. The early pharmaceutical and prescribed drug supply gave way to a huge glut of high-grade (often 30 per cent to 50 per cent purity) imported heroin. In time, police activity reduced the illegally available drug supply, causing a swing back to prescribed drugs, this time from sympathetic general practitioners and hospital doctors. In 1985 this was often buprenorphine and benzodiazepines, and the problems of the former were described early in 1986 when large numbers of individuals were found to be using this drug by injection (Robertson and Bucknall 1986). Indeed, since that time Temgesic (buprenorphine) has been the single most frequently injected drug and some younger drug users have had no experience of heroin. Sources of Temgesic included local prescriptions from general practitioners but it was also coming through prescriptions obtained from private doctors in London and resold north of the border. Awareness of this problem and the arrival of new health professionals dealing with drug users increased the amount of prescribed methadone and other non-injectable opiates subsequent to 1986.

The present situation is therefore of an actively injecting drug subculture using mainly pharmaceutically derived drugs, but also availing itself of illegally imported drugs through outlets in Glasgow and London and, on occasions, locally. The failure of a regular supply of any single drug means that most Edinburgh drug users take a variety of substances, including heroin, amphetamine, Temgesic, Diconal, cyclizine, benzodiazepines, and most recently cocaine – all by injection. Poor supplies also give rise to the occasional injection of drugs atypically favoured by drug users, such as tricyclic anti-depressants, sedatives and others.

THE EMERGENCE OF DRUG SERVICES

The preceding description may give an impression of clarity in our understanding of the Edinburgh situation. Nevertheless, it must be remembered that many pieces of the jigsaw are still missing and may remain so. The developing of the full effect of the AIDS epidemic is likely, however, to demonstrate the real numbers affected and the degree of penetration of the virus into the heterosexual community. The presence of many ill-informed infected individuals choosing to ignore their predicament is a source of anxiety for many health workers, who expect that transmission continues in some sectors by needle sharing and sexual contact. The expected morbidity and mortality due to AIDS in the forthcoming decade will give rise to increased social and domestic distress when young adults, parents and children manifest the disease.

Remembering that our knowledge at the present time pertains largely to those infected four or more years ago, people being infected today may not become clinically recognisable with HIV illness well into the 1990s. As in other places, prevention and reducing the risk of transmission are fundamental. Needle-exchange schemes (both directly funded by health boards and through general practices) have recently been sanctioned by the Scottish Office and pharmacists in some areas are now willing to sell needle and syringes to known or presumed drug users. Increased psychiatric support in the form of a community-based team supporting general practitioners is now rapidly moving the situation forward. Such workers liaise with street and voluntary agencies and provide community psychiatric nursing supervision. Hospital and social work agencies are now rapidly evolving a network of resources to provide a system to catch problems as they arise. New schemes to provide clean equipment and substitute drug prescriptions in an outreach situation are in an embryonic stage and may prove to be significant. Nevertheless, the areas of deficiency are still widespread with not one single hospital bed yet set aside specifically for the treatment of drug dependence, and there is still no residential unit able to offer detoxification and crisis intervention. Services therefore are finally emerging, if in a somewhat piecemeal fashion.

CHANGES IN SHARING BEHAVIOUR

An important change has occurred in the subculture. Accepting, in the immediate future, that drug injecting cannot be extinguished completely, it is gratifying to note a reduction in frequency of injecting and sharing of injecting equipment (Robertson *et al.* 1988a). This may be due to awareness of AIDS, an ageing and maturing drug subculture, or intervention with substitute drug prescribing. Hopefully, it is not an illusion. It is clear, however, that needle sharing still persists and that the dangers of transmission by unprotected heterosexual contact are largely ignored.

CONCLUSION

The 'Edinburgh epidemic' can only be truly described after the elapse of several more years. What is already apparent is that a huge cohort of men and women in their late teens or early twenties has been infected with the Human Immunodeficiency Virus. The final story of AIDS in Edinburgh may be one of an early rapid increase in infected drug users and perhaps a subsequent heterosexual epidemic over following decades. Drug misuse continues and new waves of users require an adequate and sensitive service designed to predict and cope with problems as they arise. The requirement for good community research cannot be overstated if it is going to be possible to increase an understanding of past events, present problems and future predictions. A better understanding is necessary of why some individuals remain well, while others – exposed in an apparently similar pattern – become HIV positive. The extent to which transmission during the epidemic years of 1983–5 was heterosexual remains an enigma and the presence of many unprotected relationships without transmission of virus holds some of the clues which could explain some of the answers to the worldwide situation. New tests such as the polymerase chain reaction (see Chapter 3) may elucidate some of the questions, but continual clear observations of behaviour are equally important.

Perhaps the most useful contribution of this case study is to present and observe events unfolding prior to the establishment of a sizeable support system for those involved with drug misuse. Observations of the natural history of a wave of drug misuse demonstrate that such epidemics probably surge and decay in a way that is to a large extent independent of treatment. The decrease in numbers of new drug users in Edinburgh appears to predate the knowledge of HIV infection and reflects the cyclical nature of drug misuse observed elsewhere (Robertson *et al.* 1988b). The corollary of this is the possibility of a further rapid increase in numbers of drug users at sometime in the future and, with HIV endemic at a high level, many problems would result. Furthermore, as has been recently observed (Des Jarlais 1988), behaviour may change in either direction and any recorded improvement in injecting technique must be sustained through continual provision of practical supports. At the present time the sheer number of drug users in some localities threatens to overwhelm enthusiastic general practitioners, pharmacists and agency workers whilst workers in other areas find little pressure. Clearly, the importance of services, properly targeted, flexible and responsive to new problems, is paramount.

REFERENCES

Advisory Council on the Misuse of Drugs (1982) *Treatment and Rehabilitation: Report of the Advisory Council on the Misuse of Drugs*, London: Department of Health and Social Services.

Advisory Council on the Misuse of Drugs (1984) *Prevention: Report of Advisory Council on the Misuse of Drugs*, London: Department of Health and Social Services.

Advisory Council on the Misuse of Drugs (1988) *AIDS and Drug Misuse Report: Part I*, London: Department of Health.

Des Jarlais, D.C. (1988) 'HIV infection among persons who inject illicit drugs: problems and progress', Stockholm: International Conference on AIDS, Keynote Address.

Ditton, A. and Speirits, K. (1982) *The Rapid Increase of Heroin Addiction in Glasgow During 1981*, University of Glasgow: Background Paper 2.

Henderson, J. (1985) Personal Communication.

Home Office (1985) *Tackling Drug Misuse: A Summary of the Government's Strategy*, London: HMSO.

Robertson, J.R. and Bucknall, A.B.V. (1986) 'Buprenorphine – dangerous drug or overlooked therapy', *British Medical Journal*, 292: 1465.

Robertson, J.R., Skidmore, C.A. and Roberts, J.J.K. (1988a) 'HIV infection in intravenous drug users: a follow-up study indicating changes in risk-taking behaviour', *British Journal of Addiction* 83: 387–91.

Robertson, J.R., Skidmore, C.A. and Roberts, J.J.K. (1988b) 'The dynamics of an illicit drug scene', *Scottish Medical Journal* 4: 293.

Stimson, G.V. and Oppenheimer, E. (1982) *Heroin Addiction: Treatment and Control in Britain*, London: Tavistock.

Ward, J.A. (1971) 'The drug scene in Scotland', *Scottish Medical Journal* 16: 376–9.

Woodside, M. (1973) 'The first 100 referrals to a Scottish drug addiction treatment centre', *British Journal of Addiction* 69: 343–55.

Chapter Ten

THE ITALIAN EPIDEMIC: A CASE STUDY

ENRICO TEMPESTA AND MASSIMO DI GIANNANTONIO

The spreading of HIV infection in Italy is characterised by features that differ greatly from those observed in other European countries. At least 68 per cent of individuals with AIDS in Italy are drug addicts who have been injecting heroin. The explanation of the difference is far from clear, but warrants particular study since Italy is one of the few countries where, for more than a decade, needles and syringes have been purchasable without restriction and at minimal cost from supermarkets which are open 24 hours per day – and yet sharing of injecting equipment appears to have been widespread.

BACKGROUND TO THE DRUG PROBLEM

Drug dependence in Italy occurred in the 1970s as an epidemic phenomenon which, in the following years, gradually evolved into an established pattern of use. Various factors such as changing cultural models and norms, a different outlook towards health policies, and a progressive change in public attitudes towards drugs, contributed to a 'social cohabitation' between the public and youthful drug user. The Surveillance Centre official data relates mainly to opiate addicts and indicates, according to data from the Ministries of Health and the Interior, numbers of between 23,200 and 33,500 individuals who turn to treatment centres seeking clinical attention per year. Although it is difficult to assess that part of the addict population which is not directly detectable, it has been estimated that the number of opiate users in Italy grew from 28,000 in 1977 to 155,000 in 1986 (an average annual increase of 23 per cent). This estimate does not take into account the abuse of other substances such as cocaine, since there is no reliable information yet available.

During this period there has been a marked increase in the availability of diversified psycho-social and psychotherapeutic services, contributing to an improvement in the quality of care available. There has also been a decrease recorded over the decade in the proportion of individuals treated with methadone in public centres (from 59 per cent to 47 per cent). There has been a simultaneous increase in the number of drug addicts undergoing protracted residential treatment in public and private therapeutic communities – from a total of 4,373 in 1983 to 7,527 individuals in 1988. The age at admission has been increasing, which suggests a progressive ageing of this population: it now has a mean age of 25.9 years.

Figure 10.1 illustrates the trend of the AIDS epidemic so far. In this respect, it should be pointed out that this trend is still growing rapidly. However, such an increase may be an overestimate, since in the last couple of years the identification standards for proven cases have been changed. Indeed, such standards now single out not only AIDS cases but AIDS Related Complex (ARC) cases as well.

The distribution according to risk groups is shown in Figure 10.2. The large representation of drug abusers is evident, as is the fact that almost all cases in women are associated with injectible drug misuse. This latter characteristic has led to the birth of 97 infants who have subsequently developed AIDS.

THE ARRIVAL OF HIV

HIV probably first appeared in Italy in 1979 in the Milan metropolitan area and one or two years later in other important Italian cities. Studies conducted on frozen serological fluids made possible the reconstruction of the HIV epidemic in Italy in different drug addict populations. Some of these blood samples were collected from people attending Public Assistance Services and under methadone treatment or at the beginning of a residential stage in therapeutic communities. This data has permitted examination of the likely date of infection, which was highest in the period between 1981 and 1984. Further samples were collected from both patients infected with hepatitis B virus and from

Figure 10.1 AIDS in Italy: reported cases

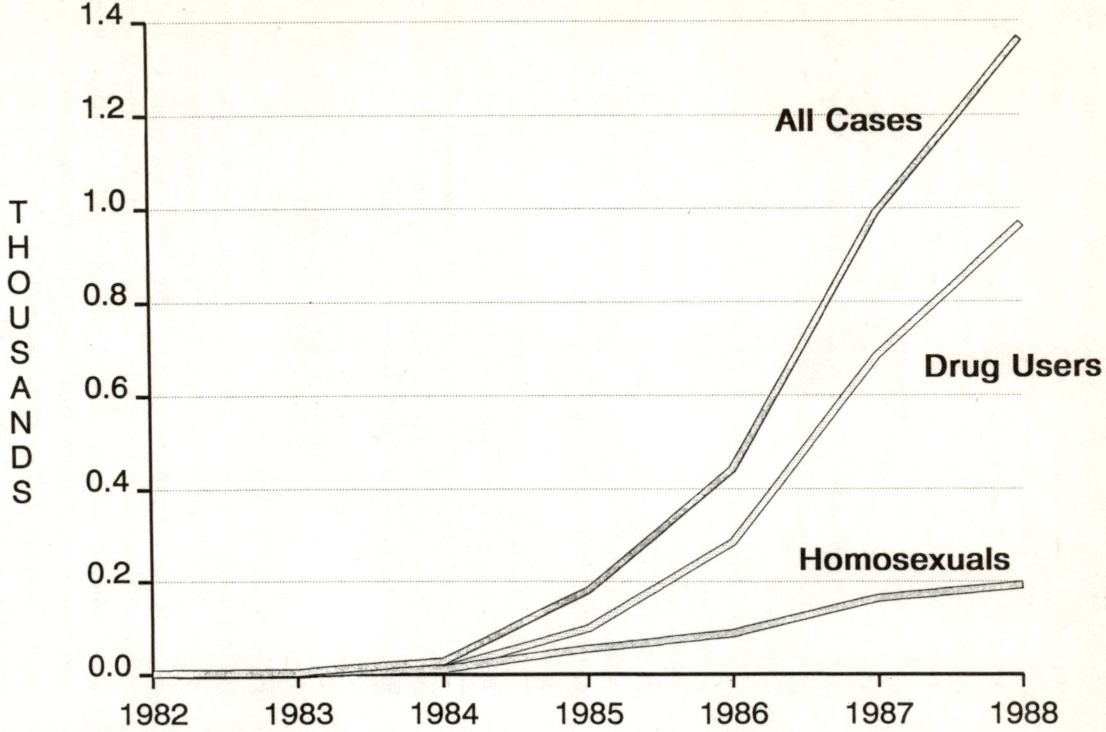

Figure 10.2 AIDS in Italy: distribution of identified risk groups

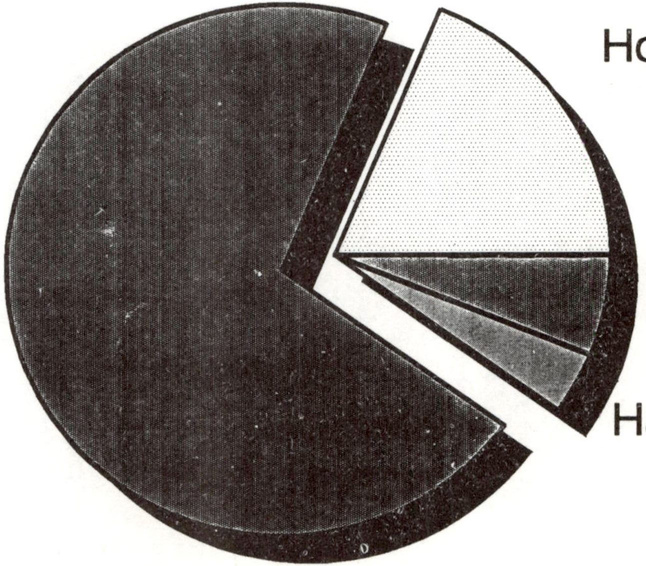

hospitalised patients. Although reliance on such samples can lead to an overestimate of the phenomenon, it is nevertheless possible to gain an understanding of the initial spread of HIV. Few samples have been available for testing from before 1978 (only 15 samples of serum were available in that year), but it seems that the virus was present from 1979 among drug addicts from the Milan area.

Between 1985 and 1987, a mass screening campaign was in progress in Italy for the identification of HIV infection in high-risk groups. A total of 52,900 subjects were tested in this period, of whom 60 per cent were drug addicts, 10 per cent homosexuals, 29 per cent other high-risk subjects (haemophiliacs, blood donors, etc.) and 1 per cent were children born from drug addict mothers (see Table 10.1). Amongst the drug addict sample, 47 per cent were found to be HIV antibody positive compared to 27 per cent found in the sample of homosexuals. (Figures given to nearest whole number.)

Table 10.1 HIV screening in an Italian risk population, 1987–9

	HIV positive	*HIV negative*	*Total*
IV drug abusers	14,882 (46.8%)	16,903 (53.2%)	31,785 (100%)
Homosexuals	1,361 (26.5%)	3,776 (73.5%)	5,137 (100%)
Children born to infected mothers	256	330	586
Other	1,422	13,970	15,392
	17,921	34,979	52,900

AIDS AND DRUG USE

It is difficult to explain the high prevalence of AIDS in injecting drug abusers, since Italy is one of the few countries where sterile syringes and needles, together with ampoules of sterilised distilled water, are available without restriction at pharmacies. The liberalisation of the sale of syringes, which may be purchased without a medical prescription, is a result of a specific health policy introduced in the mid-1970s as a preventive strategy, when public authorities were faced with fast-growing heroin abuse paralleled by an increase in the number of hepatitis B cases. Needles and syringes are readily available at low cost. For example, an insulin-type syringe costs approximately 15 pence (UK) or 20–25 cents (US). Some pharmacies have long been open 24 hours per day and it is planned that several will be open during the nights, the exact number being determined by the size of the local population. Availability of needles and syringes is, therefore, not the only factor to be taken into consideration when examining the relationship between needle sharing and the transmission of HIV infection (Weisert *et al.* 1989). Other potentially relevant factors include the following: cultural patterns of needle sharing and special patterns of behaviour, especially in the largest cities, and lack of knowledge in the past concerning the consequences of needle sharing and sexual promiscuity.

AIDS AND STUDIES OF PSYCHO-SOCIAL IMPLICATIONS IN DRUG ADDICTS

Following the HIV epidemic in Italy several changes have occurred in the behaviour of risk populations, especially in homosexual and drug addict groups. Changes in various aspects of psycho-social characteristics of drug addicts (e.g. sexual habits, consciousness of epidemic risks, knowledge of HIV transmission modalities, subjective evaluations about AIDS implications, addictive patterns) are now being monitored. Research data have been collected on 305 addicts from different Italian cities. Data were collected from hospitals, therapeutic communities and public services in an effort to achieve the widest sources possible for information.

Clinical aspects

HIV infection rates amongst populations of drug users are high (Rome, 42 per cent; Turin, 35 per cent; Milan, 53 per cent). This mainly affects those subjects with a long drug dependence history. Almost all have injected drugs (Rome, 96 per cent; Turin, 93 per cent; Milan, 97 per cent). The prevalence of Hepatitis B viral infection in the drug-using population is similar in each of the three cities studied (Rome, 52 per cent; Turin, 68 per cent; Milan, 64 per cent).

Sexual behaviour

It is rather difficult to outline a clear picture of sexual habits. None the less, studies clearly showed a rather frequent change of sexual partners. However, the most interesting and alarming finding was the difference registered in the use of condoms according to the different sexual behaviours.

In heterosexual subjects, only a very small part of the sample population (11 per cent) made use of this type of protection. In the group of bisexual subjects, however, those who were HIV positive were found to use condoms more frequently. The spreading of HIV infection and the ensuing increase of AIDS-related deaths has determined a rather alarming situation, often leading to reactions of panic among the population of drug addicts, but it seems not to be enough to modify basically the habits and sexual preferences of addicts. The role played by sexuality in HIV diffusion among drug addicts was investigated. The findings reveal an independent strong association between sex with known seropositive subjects and HIV seropositivity, and an interaction between needle sharing and sexual promiscuity in determining the spread also of other retroviral infections (HTLV-I).

Furthermore, a significant independent association has been found between male-to-male sex and HIV seropositivity. However, the proportion of male drug addicts admitting homo/bisexuality is relatively low and it is unlikely that this behaviour could be a major factor in the spread of HIV.

Subjective evaluations and awareness

The studies attempted to assess both the degree of knowledge and the type of information possessed by drug addicted subjects and to evaluate their personal experience in relation to the risk of infection and the socio-cultural models characterising the younger generations. Eighty-seven per cent of the population sampled believed themselves to be sufficiently informed as to the significance of AIDS and as to the modalities of infection. Such information was found to have been acquired mainly through the mass media (62 per cent) rather than through health care facilities.

The personal responses have confirmed both the difficulty and necessity of planning prevention campaigns presupposing different subcategories of addict populations. On the other hand, there evidently remained a large proportion of the drug addicts interviewed who gave the impression of not having been excessively concerned with the problem, or at least having adopted a fatalistic attitude. Similarly, about 40 per cent of the subjects believed that no remarkable changes had occurred in their pattern of drug use and injecting behaviours, notwithstanding the AIDS alarm.

Needle sharing

Sharing of injecting equipment is one of the highest risk factors in contracting HIV among drug addicts. According to the research data, we could hypothesise that there are two types of injectors. A first group of drug users are heavily conditioned to the ritualistic and social use of drugs in which needle sharing has a high symbolic meaning. A second group of drug users have responded to the hepatitis B epidemic in the 1970s, and have become more aware of the hygienic measures required in preparing and injecting drugs. Needle sharing and promiscuity in this second group seem to be due more to circumstantial reasons.

It is this second group that may particularly benefit from easier access to syringes. The same does not apply to the subjects belonging to the first group, for their peculiar psychopathology prevents them from being sensitive to prevention-promoting campaigns. Moreover, for this first group, every injection is a symbolic challenge to death, and the drive for drugs is stronger than any other consideration.

The sharing of needles and syringes is not the only serious problem with which we are confronted. The more we study the pattern of use and the ritual of injecting practices, the more we realise that attention should also be paid to every other aspect of preparing an injection that may cause contamination: in particular, the spoon and other tools used in preparing a dose may also be vehicles of transmission.

A research study of a sample of 180 individuals gave more detailed information on motivations determining needle sharing. Forty-eight per cent said that they shared needles because of unavailability of 'works', 9 per cent because syringe purchase presented problems, 7 per cent for habit, and only 3 per cent for lack of money. (Thirty-two per cent did not answer.) Needle sharing appeared to be very common among the drug addicts in the study. Moreover, a close association between HIV seropositivity and this practice was found, the risk increasing with the frequency of needle sharing. Surprisingly, most drug users affirmed that syringe 'unavailability' was the most important reason for not using a sterile one. However, it must be acknowledged that it is extremely difficult for a drug addict to plan his daily life and, consequently, to inject heroin safely.

It has been hypothesised that despite the provision of pharmacy sales of needles and syringes, some pharmacists might refuse to have relationships with drug users and might sometimes refuse to sell them syringes. Further, it was suggested that the cost, although low, might still deter sales. Therefore, during the last three years, several groups of different political backgrounds have put forward proposals for the free distribution of needles and syringes to drug abusers, or have proposed needle and syringe exchange programmes. These types of approach encountered major opposition from many sections of the public for ethical, medico-legal and social reasons. An important objection was the untenability of the government and regional public authorities sanctioning, in this way, an apparent 'legalisation' of behaviours such as drug use.

CONCLUSION

It seems clear that a large proportion of the drug addicts who were examined contracted the HIV infection between 1980 and 1984 when the AIDS alarm had not yet gone off in Italy. Several features of the Italian epidemic are of international interest – in particular, the apparent failure of the over-the-counter availability of needles and syringes to limit the spread of HIV amongst injecting drug addicts.

One striking aspect is the long drug addiction history of the majority of Italian drug addicts. On the one hand, this raises the problem as to the role played by opiates on the body's immune system; on the other hand, it calls for an effort to implement a secondary and tertiary prevention policy. Such a health policy should respond to the problems of this population, which is by now characterised by well-defined addictive behaviours associated with great difficulties in changing. For many drug addicts, the sharing of needles for a long time was not only felt as a 'need' but also as a way to 'communicate' with other drug addicts, and this factor is believed to have contributed to the spreading of HIV infection. This hypothesis will be further confirmed in the months and years to come by the monitoring of currently HIV-negative subjects.

REFERENCES

Tempesta, E. and Di Giannantonio, M. (1988) 'Sharing needles and the spread of HIV in Italy's addict population', in R. Battjes and W. Pickens (eds) *Needle Sharing among Intravenous Drug Abusers: National and International Perspectives*, Washington: National Institute on Drug Abuse, Research Monograph Series 80.

Weisert, A., Rossi, G.B. and Verani, P. (1989) 'Needle sharing and other behaviours related to HIV spread among intravenous drug users', *AIDS* 3: 247–8.

Part Four

RESPONDING: RETHINKING POLICY

Chapter Eleven

REVISING POLICY AND PRACTICE: NEW IDEAS ABOUT THE DRUGS PROBLEM

GERRY V. STIMSON

HIV and AIDS provide the greatest challenge yet to drug policies and services. Policy-makers and practitioners, in law enforcement, education and prevention, and in treatment and helping services, have been forced to reassess their ways of dealing with drug problems; this includes clarifying their aims, identifying their objectives and priorities for their work, their styles of working and relationships with clients, and the location of the work. Within a space of about three years, mainly between 1986 and 1988, there have been major debates about HIV, AIDS and injecting drug use. In years to come, it is likely that the late 1980s will be identified as a key period of crisis and transformation in the history of drugs policy.

It would take more than this chapter to cover all the issues, many of which are indicated in national assessments such as the report by the US Presidential Commission on the Human Immunodeficiency Virus Epidemic (1988a), the UK Advisory Council on the Misuse of Drugs reports on *AIDS and Drug Misuse* (1988, 1989), World Health Organization consultations such as the 1986 Stockholm meeting on *AIDS among Drug Abusers* (1987) and the various governmental and quasi-governmental commissions on AIDS and drug use that have been established in many countries. The aim of this chapter is therefore to attempt to identify several themes in the debate. Many of the ideas that are currently circulating have not necessarily been translated into common practice: in most countries there is a marked gap between policy debate and work-place rhetoric on the one hand, and actual practices on the other.

This chapter will step back from protagonism and proselytism; the aim is not to say what *should* be done about HIV and injectors.

Rather, it attempts to undertake a fairly detached description of current trends.

RECONCEPTUALISING THE NATURE OF THE DRUG PROBLEM

AIDS and HIV help clarify issues. One of the ways to understand the 'drug problem' is to understand the way in which societies *respond* to drug problems – and a key feature is the way in which drug problems are conceptualised: the way they are discussed, presented in scientific meetings, written about in medical textbooks, scientific articles and government reports.

This is not merely a semantic game. Our views on drug problems reflect and shape the reality they address. They have major consequences for policy and resource allocation, and real impacts on the people we are dealing with – people who use drugs. This conceptual work goes on at a ground level, but from time to time is formalised in the key committees that have been established at crisis points in the history of our relationship with drugs. In part, these conceptual transformations occur because of the elusiveness of the phenomena which are the focus of our attention. Thomas Kuhn adopted the term 'paradigm' to describe the overarching theories and frameworks that scientists use to explain the world (Kuhn 1970). The social and medical sciences have a variety of paradigms; psychoanalysis, criminology, biomedicine, marxism, and so on, may be seen as different ways of understanding and explaining the world. They make different assumptions about the nature of the social world and of human behaviour. Drug use does not fit neatly into any of the common paradigms, therefore much effort goes into arguing about what sort of problem it is. Is it, as was argued 100 years ago, a moral illness, a disease that affects the individual's will (Harding 1988)? Is it a medical problem – a disease with clear aetiology, prognosis and treatment? Is it a criminal problem, a matter for legislation and enforcement? Is it basically a moral problem – that we do not like what drug users do? Is it a social problem – a reflection of structural disadvantage and alienation? Or, to preview recent debate, is it a public health problem?

The paradigms change. This can be seen in an examination of the various paradigms of drug use circulating before HIV appeared. In the years following the first international drug control agreements (at Shanghai in 1909 and The Hague in 1912), both the USA and the UK (under the 1914 Harrison Act and the 1920 Dangerous Drugs Act) placed controls on the availability of narcotic drugs, and limited their possession to legitimate medical use. Both countries were then faced with the question whether it was legitimate for doctors to prescribe to addicts; in the USA this issue was decided in the courts – the answer was no – and thus began a period of drugs policy dominated by law enforcement which lasted through to the 1960s. In the UK the answer was yes – and thus began a period of drugs policy that was mainly medical in inspiration (though operating within a penal framework). The Rolleston Committee of 1926, which shaped British policy, is interesting because it defined the drug problem as a problem of addiction, and addiction was 'a manifestation of disease and not a mere form of vicious indulgence' (Departmental Committee on Morphine and Heroin Addiction 1926: 11). This view persisted to the 1960s, when it was replaced in the Brain Committee's deliberations by a modified medical view: the problem now was that addiction was a 'socially infectious condition' (Interdepartmental Committee on Drug Addiction 1965). The emphasis then was on the potential for the spread of drug use: a metaphorical disease, a behaviour that is spread from one person to another.

Later in the UK, as medicine itself became more 'social', and extended itself away from the hospital, the medical view was diluted, epitomised in the Advisory Council on the Misuse of Drugs definition of the 'problem drug taker' as

> Any person who experiences social, psychological, physical or legal problems related to intoxication and/or regular excessive consumption and/or dependence as a consequence of his own use of drugs or other chemical substances (excluding alcohol and tobacco).
>
> (Advisory Council on the Misuse of Drugs 1982)

This shift away from addiction to a consideration of the broad range of problems that can be associated with drug use (even in the absence of dependence) paralleled changes in professional perceptions of alcohol use: here the conceptual shift was from a concern with the addicted alcoholic, to a concern with the problem drinker and the range of problems that can occur with alcohol in the absence of addiction.

These changes in British thinking have occurred, interestingly, at a time when in the USA a more medical view of addiction as a disease has prevailed. This suggests that, internationally, different paradigms can coexist. It is also the case, of course, that different paradigms coexist within countries. In the UK the paradigm of the 'problem drug taker' coexists with the law enforcement paradigm of the 'war on drugs' which has a scenario where the main actors are 'traffickers', 'user-dealers' and 'users', each of whom exist at a different place in the demonology. The existence of these different views can confuse debate, for the key terms have meaning in the context in which they are used: for example, for one person 'prevention' may mean education programmes to discourage drug use; for a government minister responsible for law enforcement, prevention may mean strengthening penal deterrence.

HIV has simplified the debate. Rather than seeing drug use as a metaphorical disease, there is now a real medical problem associated with injecting drug use. All can agree that this is a major health problem for people who inject drugs, their sexual partners and their children. In the muddled world of drug policy, there *is* agreement about the nature and threat of HIV. Here is a clear, identifiable and measurable target. For once, government ministers, civil servants, professional advisors, practitioners in the field, can be in broad agreement. In the UK, for example, the government has in recent years pushed through health and social policies which have often been opposed by many professional workers. But the drugs field, since the advent of HIV, has been marked by a lack of conflict and criticism about aims, objectives and strategies. Such consensus is rare in the UK, and probably not found in the USA, where there is consensus about the new aims of drug policies, but considerable disagreement about objectives and strategies.

PROTECTING THE PUBLIC HEALTH AND THE PUBLIC PURSE

It is hard to know whether this new concern for the drug injector arises from altruistic concern for the drug user *per se*, or from concern with the threat posed by the drug injector to the health of others, or whether it is a concern about the resource implications of treating drug injectors who develop AIDS.

Few policy documents avoid mention of the broader threat to public health or public resources. The US Presidential Commission points out that:

> Our nation's ability to control the course of the HIV epidemic depends greatly on our ability to control the problem of intravenous drug abuse. Intravenous and other drug abuse is a substantial carrier for infection, a major port of entry for the virus into the larger population.
>
> (Presidential Commission on the Human Immunodeficiency Virus Epidemic, 1988a: 94)

The document also addresses the resource implications, and mentions the 'staggering costs of providing health care for drug abusers with AIDS' (1988b). Certainly, one effect of such appeals is to draw public attention to the very real problems faced by the potential spread of HIV infection, and legitimise the expenditure of funds on an unpopular and undeserving group, and one that is often seen as suffering from a self-inflicted malady.

The emergence of pragmatism

The new public health model of HIV and drug use is marked by pragmatism. In the UK it is interesting that Conservative health ministers, with support from ministerial colleagues, and the enthusiasm of civil service and other advisors, have pursued a pragmatic rather than a moralistic policy. As one minister put it, it is not a matter for dogma but for hard, practical common sense. It is easy to envisage an alternative scenario where the main thrust was moral condemnation of the undeserving (gays and junkies); with an appeal to self-restraint, celibacy, family values, and simple conventional pleasures. (An interesting issue is how a Conservative government came to pursue such a pragmatic policy on AIDS.)

DRUG USE, HIV AND THE THREAT TO PUBLIC HEALTH

At one level the prevention of HIV transmission between and from injectors appears easy; preventing people from injecting drugs also prevents the spread of the virus: if people are helped to avoid injecting drugs in the first place, or helped to stop injecting them, then the HIV risk is avoided. But the world of drug use is not so simply changed: preventive education, penal deterrence and treatment to help people become abstinent, all have an extremely dismal impact on the prevalence of drug problems. Given what is known about what works (and what does not) in drug prevention and treatment, it is unrealistic to expect that in the short term fewer people will start injecting, or that large numbers of injectors will stop using drugs.

A starting-point for the public health model is the premise that countries with drug injectors will have many people who are currently unable and unwilling to stop injecting. The pool of current injectors has been put at 1.2 million in the US, at between 750,000 and 1 million in Europe (World Health Organization 1988), and at between 37,000 and 75,000 in the UK (Advisory Council on the Misuse of Drugs 1988). The analysis therefore suggests that these people are an urgent target for the prevention of HIV transmission.

A key issue in shaping drug policies is the choice that has been posed between two targets – between the prevention of HIV transmission and the prevention of drug abuse. Some policy debates have now put the prevention of HIV higher on the agenda than the prevention of drug problems (the latter for now either abandoned as a hopeless task, or relegated to secondary importance in face of the immediate public health issue).

The clarity of the new public health view on drug problems is found in the UK, parts of Europe and Australia. The report on *AIDS and Drug Misuse* states:

> We have no hesitation in concluding that the spread of HIV is a greater danger to individual and public health than drug misuse.
>
> (Advisory Council on the Misuse of Drugs 1988: 17)

A similar view is put, in more diplomatic terms, by the World Health Organization (1987: 9)

> The relative risks of drug abuse and HIV infection must be carefully weighed. On balance, those of HIV infection will generally be found to be the more serious. Policies aimed at

> drug reduction must therefore not be allowed to prejudice measures taken against these risks.

In this paradigm, prevention takes on yet a further meaning – the key prevention task is not the prevention of drug use, but the prevention of HIV infection and transmission.

THE NEW VIEW OF THE DRUG USER, POLICY AND PRACTICE

What is now required is an analysis of this new public health paradigm of drug problems. As with earlier paradigms, it comprises ideas about the nature of the drug user, the nature of the problem, the nature of the task, the people appropriate to deal with the task and the place from which they should work, and their relationships with clients.

First, ideas about the nature of the drug user are shifting. The focus is not on the problem drug taker *per se*, but on the problem drug user who injects drugs. The new conception of the injector is at variance with many earlier views about the nature of the drug user and injector. The drug injector is now seen as a rational actor, who will respond to public health information. The drug injector is seen as having a new concern for his or her health – whilst they might wish to inject dangerous drugs, they are willing to act in such a way as to prevent their risk of HIV infection. The injector is also seen as able to engage in rational health management and behaviour, and balance long-term threats to health against short-term pleasures (see Chapter 14).

Second, the nature of the problem has altered. The body, and relationships between bodies, has become the focus for social intervention, rather than the mind (Lart 1988), and the leading ideological framework is health promotion, harm minimisation, risk reduction and, in Holland, the 'normalisation' of drug problems. As expressed in the Advisory Council on the Misuse of Drugs report (1988: 17):

> We must therefore be prepared to work with those who continue to misuse drugs to help them reduce the risks involved in doing so, and above all the risk of acquiring or spreading HIV.

This view is also found in the US Presidential Commission on the Human Immunodeficiency Virus Epidemic, which supports the argument for the safer use of injecting equipment in those who persist in injecting.

The harm-minimisation approach echoes the safer-sex campaigns which started with gay men and subsequently extended to the heterosexual population. Put simply, people will not want to abstain from sexual activity, therefore they must be encouraged to engage in safer sex. The idea has now been extended to drug injectors – if they won't stop injecting, they should and could inject drugs in a safer way.

Third, the nature of the work also changes in this new paradigm. Out go confrontation and coercion, and making services available only to the deserving and the motivated. The lack of resources for the treatment of drug problems in the UK in the 1970s and 1980s began a trend to shorter-term contract prescription of methadone. Queues were used to test clients' motivation. In consequence, only a minority of referrals for treatment actually passed through all the 'hurdles' and were accepted for treatment (Love and Gossop 1985). This has now been turned around – the emphasis is now on reaching people and making treatment and other services more accessible, with an open-door policy. One of the key recommendations of the US Presidential Commission is to make treatment available on demand. The commission estimates that in the USA this will require at least 2,500 new drug abuse treatment facilities, and 59,000 new drug abuse treatment workers.

Out go big targets – such as abstinence; in come smaller targets, goals which fall short of abstinence (see Chapter 19). Out go single goals; in comes a hierarchy of goals – ranging from becoming drug free, switching from injecting to oral use, a decrease in drug use, and avoiding sharing needles and syringes. The task is to 'nudge' and 'tickle' the injector through the small changes that they will accept, which may be of cumulative significance in changing individual behaviour and reducing collective risk of HIV.

Fourth, ideas about who is equipped to do work, and where they should work, are changing. There are two strands to this. On the one hand, the new emphasis on health is forcing a partial remedicalisation of the work: psychiatrists are having to relearn physical medicine and conduct medical examinations; nurses are considered good at harm minimisation; all drug workers are urged to acquaint themselves with knowledge of physical aspects of HIV infection. On the other hand, the problem is to reach as many injectors as possible in the time available. Services can be changed to improve their attractiveness, but this still leaves those who are unwilling or unable to present themselves. Services therefore must go out into the community to reach the injector, and, if possible, help change drug cultures by enabling mutual organisation and help. This task requires community workers, outreach workers and the enrolment of ex-addicts (and in some cases present drug takers) as health educators.

Fifth, the changes suppose a changed relationship between the professional worker and client. It is no longer a matter of the client as supplicant for a scarce service, given only on the terms and conditions set by the professional worker. Drug injectors cannot be forced to use a service or to like the service that is offered. This suggests the development of a more co-operative and egalitarian model of the relationship. This involves enticing injectors through 'user-friendly' services, by making services more acceptable, with staff 'enabling' and 'empowering' injectors to change their behaviour by providing them with the information and promoting motivation to change, and the means to make those changes (methadone, syringes, condoms).

CONCLUSION

Bound up, as we all are, in these major attempts to rethink drug policies and practice in the light of HIV, we lack the benefit of historical distancing and hindsight which facilitates our attempts to analyse previous periods in drug policy. As presented here, these new ideas appear as a distinct break with earlier ones, but as with many conceptual and practical changes, the possibilities are inherent in earlier ideas and work. It is perhaps a matter of emphasis and direction, rather than abrupt rupture with the recent past.

When we look back on this period in 10 or 20 years' time, how much of what has been identified here will have been turned into practice and have had real consequences for drug injectors and the broader public? For how long will agencies and their staff be able to sustain this new image of the drug user, when (to be realistically pessimistic) they will be faced with recalcitrant injectors who do not change their behaviour? Will the public health model come to be perceived as a failure, to be replaced by a re-emergent law enforcement model? How acceptable will these policies and practices appear when there are substantial numbers of HIV-positive sick injectors? How much concern will there be for the injector if the epidemic becomes established in heterosexual populations?

Such speculations must for now be put on hold. Earlier in this chapter it was claimed that analysing the way we respond to drugs is not merely a semantic game. It is important to step back in order to grasp the direction in which current policy and practice are developing. This is not just of sociological and historial interest. The stakes are high: if the paradigm turns out to be wrong or ineffectual, the consequences are potentially disastrous.

REFERENCES

Advisory Council on the Misuse of Drugs (1982) *Treatment and Rehabilitation*, London: Department of Health and Social Security.

Advisory Council on the Misuse of Drugs (1988) *AIDS and Drug Misuse Report: Part I*, London: Department of Health.

Advisory Council on the Misuse of Drugs (1989) *AIDS and Drug Misuse Report: Part II*, London: Department of Health.

Departmental Committee on Morphine and Heroin Addiction (1926) *Report*, London: HMSO.

Harding, G. (1988) *Opiate Addiction, Morality and Medicine: From Moral Illness to Pathological Disease*, London: Macmillan.

Interdepartmental Committee on Drug Addiction (1965) *Second Report*, London: HMSO.

Kuhn, T.S. (1970) *Structure of Scientific Revolutions*, Chicago: University of Chicago Press.

Lart, R.A. (1988) Personal Communication.

Love, J. and Gossop, M. (1985) 'The processes of referral and disposal within a London drug dependence clinic', *British Journal of Addiction* 80: 435–40.

Presidential Commission on the Human Immunodeficiency Virus Epidemic (1988a) *Report*, Washington.

Presidential Commission on the Human Immunodeficiency Virus Epidemic (1988b) *AIDS commission releases chairman's recommendations*, Washington.

World Health Organization (1987) *AIDS among Drug Abusers*, Copenhagen: World Health Organization Regional Office.

World Health Organization (1988) 'Meeting on drug intervention strategies and HIV infection: preliminary consensus statement', Geneva: World Health Organization.

Chapter Twelve

AIDS AND INJECTING DRUG USE IN AUSTRALIA: A CASE STUDY IN POLICY DEVELOPMENT AND IMPLEMENTATION

ALEX WODAK

IN THE BEGINNING

For many countries, the recognition of the existence of AIDS in 1981 came too late. In these countries, tens of thousands of male homosexuals, injecting drug users and haemophiliacs were already infected and the national blood supply was already contaminated before the alarm bells began ringing. The goal of national AIDS policies from then on could only be to slow down the further spread of infection within and from these groups and to care for those already infected. Each country in turn recognising the magnitude of its own national problem then joined the international cargo cult waiting for the arrival of effective treatment and vaccine.

Australia also succumbed to this by now familiar pattern. As in most western countries, homosexual/bisexual men were the first group to be infected. Sydney, the largest Australian city with a population of 3.5 million, has always had a large homosexual community and an identifiable homosexual area in the inner city. The pilgrimage to the San Francisco gay scene had long been part of the Sydney homosexual identity and ensured that the gay ghetto in Sydney would be the epicentre for the AIDS epidemic in Australia.

In this chapter, Australia is examined as a case study to try and determine which factors assisted and which retarded the development of effective AIDS prevention policies for drug users. The purpose of this exercise is to extract lessons which could be applied to other countries although recognising that the response of each country must be seen from within the context of its own national perspective and social conditions.

At the beginning of the century, with the recent development of a federal system of government, Australia was a progressive and enlightened country with a per capita income among the highest in the world. By the early 1980s, Australia, still a prosperous country, was pursuing middle of the road economic and social policies. Relative to international standards, Australia's response to the AIDS epidemic has been pragmatic and prompt and the policy response to HIV infection in injecting drug users is no exception. This case study is complicated by the federal structure of Australian politics whereby a central Commonwealth government shares power with six states and two territories. The Commonwealth Department of Community Services and Health occupies a position of leadership in relation to health departments of states and territories. Although uniformity of policies and implementation is a rarity, across jurisdictions some degree of common ground is usually evident.

NEVER SEND TO KNOW FOR WHOM THE BELL TOLLS . . .

By October 1988, Australia ranked sixth among OECD countries in terms of AIDS cases per head of population with 2.1 cases per 100,000. Homosexual/bisexual males constituted 88 per cent of the first 1,000 cases of AIDS with homosexual/bisexual male injecting drug users comprising an additional 2.5 per cent and heterosexual injecting drug users a further 0.6 per cent. These figures are remarkable on two counts. First, Australia has so far had relatively few cases of AIDS in injecting drug users. Almost all western countries badly affected by HIV infection, except Australia and Canada, have had a far higher proportion of AIDS cases among injecting drug users. In both Spain and Italy, injecting drug users have constituted over half the national AIDS cases. In the United States, from the beginnings of the epidemic, homosexual/bisexual male drug users have comprised 8 per cent of AIDS cases, with heterosexual injecting drug users representing an additional 17 per cent. Second, it is remarkable that Australia does not have a far higher incidence of AIDS in drug users as the epicentre of the Australian epidemic is also the area in Sydney most strongly associated with the drug subculture.

It is possible that injecting drug users have not figured prominently in the Australian cases reported thus far because there are relatively few drug users to become infected. Although estimation of the number of injecting drug users in a community is beset with problems of definition and methodology, on available data, Australia has a higher prevalence of injecting drug users than the Netherlands or the United Kingdom, but far less than the United States. It is also possible that there is a far higher incidence of AIDS in Australian drug users than presently reported but the system of classification of AIDS cases could be subject to consistent and so far undetected bias. However, the rate of HIV infection in Australian drug users also appears low and is consistent with the low incidence of AIDS in injecting drug users in the country. The possibility of large numbers of injecting drug users succumbing to complications of HIV infection before developing manifestations meeting the diagnostic criteria for AIDS is also not supported by existing data, even though this development has already been reported in New York City. It is tempting to ascribe the phenomenon of limited HIV infection in Australian drug users to clear-sighted policy formulation and vigorous implementation, denying any possible contribution from luck.

HIV AND INJECTING DRUG USERS IN AUSTRALIA: THE EVOLUTION OF A POLICY RESPONSE

In 1985, the major medical and scientific body established in Australia to advise the Commonwealth government on AIDS, the National AIDS Task Force, publicly advocated increasing the availability of sterile needles and syringes to reduce the spread of infection in injecting drug users. Early in 1985 a Sydney group of past and present drug users, together with health professionals, attempted to set up a self-help organisation called the AIDS Drugs Information Collective (ADIC). Unsuccessful attempts were made to obtain government funding over the next two years. In late 1986 the National Advisory Committee on AIDS (NACAIDS) established an IVDU Working Party (including a representative of the target population) and similar advisory committees were established by several state health departments at the time. Strategic plans began to evolve and attempts to increase the availability of sterile needles and syringes were the major preoccupation. From these times, expert advisors were often divided by their emphasis on the need to provide politically palatable solutions. A minority view advocated maintaining a role of pristine scientific expertise with all implementation questions left for elected officials.

The introduction of needle and syringe exchange schemes

The implementation of a pilot needle and syringe scheme in November 1986 by a group of Sydney alcohol and drug workers marked a turning-point. Advisory committees had agonised over taking the momentous first step and deliberated on how best to monitor and evaluate the effectiveness of such a programme. The pilot programme was in breach of recently proclaimed legislation but no prosecution or police action was undertaken.

In December 1986 the New South Wales Department of Health, previously opposed to increasing the availability of sterile needles and syringes, announced the introduction of a needle and syringe distribution scheme through retail pharmacies. Within 18 months, all jurisdictions bar one (covering a population of 400,000) had started distribution or exchange of sterile needles and syringes. By 1988, the State of New South Wales (population 5.5 million) had approved 40 needle and syringe exchange outlets and 300 retail pharmacies were distributing needles and syringes with some in addition providing exchange. Approximately 1.5 million sterile needle and syringes were exchanged or distributed in 1988 in New South Wales alone, with official estimates indicating the existence of 10,000–14,000 injecting drug users in the state.

The development of treatment services

Expansion of drug treatment services had begun in 1985 but received impetus nationally in 1986 with the initiation of a National Campaign Against Drug Abuse (NCADA) providing 100 million Australian dollars in funding over a three-year period. The principal aim of the NCADA was the minimisation of harm consequent on drug use. Reduction of drug use was seen as a means to an end, but not an end in itself. The NCADA was a critical factor in the response to HIV infection. First, the identification of harm reduction as the principal aim of national drug policies subsequently facilitated the synthesis of HIV containment policies with national drug policies. Second, the expansion and improvement in drug treatment facilities, data collection, training and research prepared the base from which a later change in goals could be effected.

In 1985 admission to methadone maintenance programmes was liberalised in New South Wales to allow the admission of HIV-infected drug users on public health grounds alone, even in the absence of criteria required for other patients. Although few drug users were admitted on this criterion alone, the change in policy was indicative of a pragmatic mood. Within the next few years, drug treatment in general and methadone maintenance programmes in particular were trebled in capacity and liberalised.

The major national policy responses to HIV infection in injecting drug users have been a series of documents prepared by the NACAIDS (subsequently the Australian National Council on AIDS) IVDU Working Party and a National AIDS Strategy Green Paper which was published in 1988. These policy documents contain a range of strategies and emphasise the need for HIV containment as a priority even above the desire to reduce illicit drug use.

Emerging debate about drug control policy

Increasingly frequent calls for drug policy reform have been heard in Australia following the implementation of needle and syringe exchanges. Although drug policy reform is still a minority view, it is gaining increasing support from many quarters including senior and distinguished public figures. Public opinion polls in 1987 and 1988 have reflected a more sceptical attitude to the efficacy of law enforcement and supported a more positive attitude to drug policy reform as a necessary response to the threat of AIDS. Cautious encouragement of an emerging debate on drug policy has been provided by the Commonwealth government.

Although a range of pragmatic strategies to contain HIV infection in injecting drug users has been clearly articulated, it should not be understood that these have been adopted and implemented with alacrity and without opposition. Australia's record may compare favourably with many other western countries, but the real criteria against which policies should be measured are the characteristics of the Human Immunodeficiency Virus and projections of the likely impact of the HIV infection on society.

FACTORS ASSISTING CHANGE

The influence of individuals

It is tempting to attribute the support for the development and implementation of relatively pragmatic policies to a few key individuals. There can be little doubt that Australia was exceedingly fortunate to have a politician with a strong record on civil liberties and humanitarian leanings as Minister for Health during the critical early years of the AIDS epidemic. The Australian emphasis on regional and international responsibilities in responding to HIV infection is consistent with the minister's personality and outlook. There can be little doubt that most other ministers who could have been the Minister for Health at the time would have supported a more conservative response to AIDS generally. It is also tempting to point to key advisors who may have had a far greater understanding of the dimensions of AIDS in the early days because of personal factors.

During the lead up to the election campaign of 1985, it became public knowledge that the Prime Minister's daughter had serious drug problems. None the less, in 1987, the wife of the Prime Minister clearly articulated her support for pragmatic approaches to HIV prevention in injecting drug users, recognising the need to minimise the harmful consequences of youthful experimentation. Various politicians with differing degrees of personal involvement in the HIV epidemic also supported the adoption of a pragmatic approach.

Whilst not denying the importance of key individuals, it is unlikely that these admirable politicians and their advisors are the entire explanation, and ascribing support for pragmatic policies to individuals simply begs the question as to how they came to be influential in the first place.

The influence of advisory bodies

Part of the explanation lies with the structuring of a series of advisory bodies with participants drawn from medicine, behavioural sciences and at-risk group representatives. These groups could not be expected to ignore entirely the extraordinary opportunity for self-promotion and aggrandisement when placed in the spotlight of AIDS. Some of the community groups, with recent memories of longstanding discrimination, could not resist the temptation of newly granted power to redress old grievances. However, a system of checks and balances has evolved not too dissimilar from the political balance between executive, legislature and judiciary. Community groups have argued that AIDS is too important to be left to the biomedical establishment. Experience has shown that community groups are also less than omniscient. Exclusion of community groups undoubtedly reduces the effectiveness of policy development and implementation although their inclusion in the process is not without its own costs. Overall, the balancing of interest groups has worked well. The establishment of parliamentary liaison groups has also fostered a bipartisan approach and forestalled the development of politically motivated responses. The AIDS policy arena in Australia has attracted an extraordinary range of talents and hard-working individuals. Although conflict has inevitably occurred, and often been publicly damaging, a harmonious sense of common purpose has been more characteristic.

The influence of media portrayal

The special role of the media was appreciated early in the epidemic and the media have been skilfully exploited and have become increasingly supportive. This has been particularly the case in regard to the response to HIV infection in injecting drug users. In the mid-1980s at the start of the NCADA, the prevailing media image of drug users was of psychopathic villains. Within a few years, more sympathetic portraits were common with increasing attention directed to the complex nature of drug use and the deficiencies of the treatment system. The villain had become, at least in part, a victim. This change was essential to generate public support for some controversial items.

The influence of government

The federal structure has been a surprising ally in the promotion of change. As more enlightened states introduced progressive policies, the more conservative states were sucked into the vortex, albeit at a slower pace. The number and range of responsible authorities, so often a barrier to progress, actually contributed to change.

The influence of research projects

A number of key research projects have also proved to be influential. These projects often owed their inspiration to the desire to provide data for determination of policies. Preliminary results were often made available to senior bureaucrats prior to publication in order to facilitate the process of decision-making.

FACTORS HINDERING CHANGE

Knowledge, attitude and – crucially – behaviour

It is often incorrectly assumed that an improvement in knowledge is a necessary precondition for attitudinal change which must occur before behaviour change. The reality is unfortunately more complex than this simple paradigm.

Injecting drug users in Australia became well informed about the AIDS epidemic relatively early. Evidence of behaviour change is not available as repeated measures studies have not been conducted. It appears that many drug users perceived that their drug-using colleagues were at risk while denying that their own needle sharing and sexual practices placed them (or their partners) at risk.

Management and worker resistance

The process of change in knowledge, attitude and risk-taking behaviour (in terms of policy support) occurred far more slowly at middle-management level. Often the greatest resistance to change came from drug and alcohol workers who prided themselves as 'agents of change' with their clients. The fear of adaptation had multiple causes including: entrenched philosophical allegiance to the disease concept; concern that past training would be irrelevant in the new public health era; and anxiety that the industrial implications of a new public health focus would result in less attractive remuneration and employment conditions.

One of the obstacles to change has a more pernicious origin.

Prevention of HIV infection in injecting drug users was for many years not accepted as a legitimate part of a health employee's role. For those involved in this lonely work in the early years there were powerful disincentives, including at times acrimonious receptions from erstwhile colleagues.

Fear of political isolation

Another theme running through the responses has been the issue of timing. Politicians and their advisors were concerned not to stray too far ahead of the flock, although the evidence from opinion polls sometimes indicated that they may have been leading from behind. The desire to reach the 'right' policies at the 'right' time has delayed many a policy which the public could well have tolerated earlier.

Dispute between government departments

A problem from the earliest days is the negative influence of government departments outside the health area. The Police and Corrective Services department cannot be expected to share the same goals and aspirations as health staff. Nor have these departments been ready to review the changing perception of drug users from archetypal villain to lynchpin of an ominous and growing public health threat. As government departments operate relatively independently, it has been difficult even to organise interdepartmental structures to facilitate communication. These difficulties have contributed to delays in revision or repeal of legislation which have slowed the implementation and reduced the effectiveness of needle and syringe exchange.

The need to review national drug policies has also suffered from the fact that the area lies outside the direct responsibilities of the health domain and is perceived as part of the bedrock of society. Consideration of the issue has been therefore ignored, avoided and postponed. It is only now that it has come into central focus.

SUMMARY

In comparison with other western countries, Australia has a relatively high incidence of AIDS per capita but infection in injecting drug users has occurred later than in many other countries despite the fact that the epicentre for the epidemic in homosexual/bisexual men lies in an area associated with drug use and injecting. To some extent this can be explained by the early adoption and vigorous implementation of pragmatic policies. However, it is harder to establish why such policies have been introduced relatively early in Australia. Undoubtedly, a few key individuals deserve enormous credit although this is a necessary but not sufficient explanation.

The success in maintaining a politically bipartisan approach has no doubt also contributed. Australia has also been relatively successful in dealing with policy development and implementation advice from biomedical, behavioural science and community groups. However, change has also required support for controversial policies from the entire community. Skilful exploitation of direct and indirect media coverage has been a consistent feature of the Australian response to AIDS. Australia was exceedingly fortunate in being able to capitalise on the fruits of a recent National Campaign Against Drug Abuse by converting some of the gains into strategies to contain HIV infection in injecting drug users. Nevertheless, many factors have delayed and obstructed change, including entrenched treatment philosophies, irreconcilable differences in priorities, industrial problems and interdepartmental sharing of responsibilities. In this regard, the case study of Australia stands as an example of both vision and intransigence, and of both success and failure.

Chapter Thirteen

THE ROLES OF PRESCRIBING

JOHN STRANG

What is it about prescribing that so enduringly attracts debate and attention? No doubt it is partly because prescribing the drug of actual misuse (or a closely related substitute) to a drug taker might reasonably be seen as merely institutionalising the drug-taking behaviour. On the other hand, it may be argued that other benefits could be accrued by such institutionalisation or that other changes may occur in its wake; if so, then it should be possible to identify these in advance, thus enabling the patient, the doctor and any observer to gauge the rate of progress towards this second-level goal. As an illustration, if the prescribing of oral methadone to an injecting heroin addict is being considered because it may help the move away from injecting and the severing of links with drug-using acquaintances, then these should be included as measures of the effectiveness of the intervention rather than just observing whether or not the drug taker is grateful for (and takes) the methadone.

Over the years there have been various waves of fashion about prescribing drugs to drug addicts; and here we are, apparently going back to what we abandoned several years ago. However, the prescribing of today cannot be considered as just the same as the prescribing of yesterday or tomorrow: rather, what is required is a consideration of today's prescribing in today's new paradigm. In steering a safe path through today's troubled, uncharted waters, we would be well advised to look at similar journeys which have been made in earlier times to see whether there are lessons which can be learned – lessons which may be capable of interpretation in the light of today's circumstances so as to give guidance in choosing the most appropriate course.

'Flexibility' is currently 'in'. This refers to the moulding of the treatment (including prescribing) to the individual characteristics of the particular patient. However, 'flexibility' has sometimes been used as a justification for indiscriminate prescribing in which the doctor moves towards a position of just prescribing on request in the naive belief that the patient should be given the authority to select the instrument from the doctor's armamentarium. Although a wider range of prescribing options may increase the potential effectiveness of therapeutic interventions, it also increases the potential for error.

The putative overall benefit of different prescribing options can be considered by use of a cost–benefit analysis or pay-off matrix. Thus, the potential advantages and disadvantages of high-threshold and low-threshold treatment programmes might appear as in Table 13.1. The recent introduction of low-threshold treatment programmes has been accompanied by increased uptake of the service and an appeal to drug users earlier in their careers, but it has simultaneously stressed the system with the increased workload and may also have facilitated relapse by the over-ready recommencement of a prescription during times of post-detoxification crisis.

Table 13.1 Pay-off matrix of high-threshold versus low-threshold prescribing programmes

	Possible advantages	*Possible disadvantages*
High-threshold	– Confirmed cases – Low spillage on to blackmarket – Ease of operation of service	– Late contact – Lost opportunities – Low penetration of wider target population
Low-threshold	– Increased uptake – Earlier contact – Good image on the street	– Prescribing to non-addicts – Facilitating relapse – Increased workload

One of the uncomfortable realities for the medical profession is that as the extent of potential prescribing is increased (and as the potential abuses of this prescribing increase), so it becomes necessary to introduce self-regulatory and/or external controls.

We need a framework which is more sophisticated than one which simply indicates whether prescribing options A, B and C should or should not exist; it must also give us some indication as to the contexts in which the different prescribing responses are appropriate. Thus, there are circumstances (see p.149) in which the prescribing of injectable drugs such as heroin or methadone ampoules might be appropriate, but it would be a travesty of the concept of flexible treatment if this was seen as a legitimate rationale for the open-handed prescribing of heroin to all and sundry.

In the next section of this chapter, an examination will be made of different specific roles which may be fulfilled by prescribing.

Prescribing for relief of withdrawal

This is probably the most straightforward application of methadone prescribing to opiate addicts. The only UK study which has compared out-patient and in-patient detoxification found significantly lower rates of achieving abstinence in the out-patient cohort (Gossop *et al.* 1986). American DARP studies of different opiate treatment modalities found 'drug treatment only' withdrawal programmes of less than 90 days to be significantly worse in terms of compliance and achievement of abstinence (Simpson and Sells 1983). The doctor considering short-term prescribing to help the addict out over the next few days should give careful thought to the longer-term treatment plan. It may be that this could prove an opportunity to engage the addict in treatment which might lead to early beneficial change, but on the other hand the practitioner must take care to avoid inadvertently prescribing maintenance by default.

The prescription as bait to capture the drug taker

Perhaps it seems paradoxical to prescribe drugs of abuse as part of the management of drug addiction; and yet on the other hand it could be such an obvious strategy for increasing the consumer appeal of the treatment programme (see Chapter 19). There is little point in having a highly effective treatment programme if no addict utilises the treatment.

One way of viewing some of our services (including the

prescribing of drugs) might be to regard them as loss-leaders. In marketing, a company may put out below-cost or even free items so as to engage the interest of a wider potential purchasing group. Similarly, pharmaceutical drug companies may arrange free lunches for medical practitioners or may sponsor independent conferences. It is important to realise that the measure of the effectiveness of the loss-leader is *not* the extent of uptake of the loss-leader itself, but is the extent of progression to the *next* step: how many of the individuals who have taken up the below-cost offer have also gone on to purchase other profit-generating items, and how many of the doctors who have received a free lunch have subsequently altered their prescribing habits? If it is to be effective, the loss-leader must be attractive in its own right, but must be of such a nature that it does not obstruct flow on to the next level at which the sought-after behaviour might occur. Low-threshold prescribing programmes or the provision of other benefits (e.g. free legal aid or needles and syringes) might be regarded as loss-leaders; thus, one measure of their value would be the extent to which they encouraged recruitment and subsequent flow on to the next level in the journey of treatment.

The prescription as adhesive to improve retention

If a particular treatment is thought to be effective, then the patient must be exposed to the treatment for a sufficient length of time for it to exert its beneficial effect. Almost without exception, treatment programmes for drug addicts are beset with problems of progressive drop-out. The particular challenge is to look for ways in which we might reduce the extent to which such drop-out occurs. Retention in treatment programmes is assuming greater importance in that it provides a mechanism whereby regular monitoring of physical status can be undertaken and whereby new anti-HIV treatments could be made available promptly as and when they become available.

The continued prescribing of drugs increases the likelihood of continued attendance – especially when the prescribed drugs are of a substance, form and dose which increases their appeal to the drug taker. A careful cost–benefit analysis will be required if a balance is to be achieved between the relative benefits and costs of longer-term prescribing regimens.

The prescription as promoter of change

The process of change is described in Chapter 19. How might the prescription have an influence on flow through this process? First, it might attract 'unmotivated' drug users into treatment so that they are available for monitoring of their ongoing HIV status and are also available for HIV treatment. However, having 'captured' the drug taker, it then becomes necessary to implement approaches which might bring about beneficial change in the precise nature of any ongoing drug use.

During the 1980s, UK drug services have tended to concentrate on the provision of abstinence-orientated programmes so that the sought-after beneficial change in drug-taking status has been obvious. However, in the changed circumstances of today, other benefits might be identified which relate to the personal and public health threat from HIV.

The concept of intermediate goals was recently introduced into the UK debate by the report on *AIDS and Drug Misuse* by the Advisory Council on the Misuse of Drugs (ACMD) (1988). At the heart of the debate about the feasibility of intermediate goals is the controversy about the nature of drug dependence itself. If the addict's drug-taking is an all-or-nothing phenomenon, then no benefit will be accrued from pursuit of some half-way goal of reduction in dose or movement away from injecting. If the drug addict is on a slippery slope from which the only escape route is complete abstinence, then discussions of reducing dose, cutting back on injecting or moderating the extent of use will merely encourage the drug taker to consider unrealistic options. On the other hand, if the addict's drug-taking behaviour is seen as malleable, then it might be possible to work towards less ambitious short-term goals which could then be seen as intermediate goals in the longer journey of treatment. Data are now emerging indicating the considerable extent to which opiate addicts are able to bring about beneficial changes in their continued drug use even though the changes fall short of abstinence itself. If treatment is seen as working through a cascade of processes of change (either sequentially or simultaneously) with the end state of each process acting as one of a hierarchy of goals, then the beneficial impact of the prescription could be gauged according to its effectiveness in achieving these intermediate goals. Some of the intermediate goals within the cascade or hierarchy might reasonably be seen as particularly important, such as the cessation of sharing injecting equipment, and the move from injectable to oral-only drug use.

The prescription as an obstructor of change

If the prescribing of drugs to a drug addict might be seen as a promoter of change in some circumstances, then might it have the opposite effect in another set of circumstances? Might it actually obstruct change that would otherwise have come about? Some of the small number of UK opiate addicts who have been in receipt of prescriptions continuously since the NHS clinics opened 20 years ago describe the provision as a mixed blessing. They explain that although they may have been at increased risk of drug-related illness or death, they might also have been more likely to have become drug-free in the absence of a continuous prescription. The out-patient comparison between injectable heroin maintenance and oral methadone maintenance conducted by Hartnoll *et al.* (1980) is interesting in this regard. It appeared that injectable heroin maintenance supported the drug-taking status quo, while the refusal to prescribe injectables and the offer of oral methadone maintenance instead appeared to cause a polarisation of the population: more did well, more did worse and fewer occupied the middle ground than in the heroin maintenance group.

The second report on *AIDS and Drug Misuse* from the ACMD (1989) considers the possible benefits that may result from the short-term prescribing of injectable drugs as an intermediate goal in carefully selected patients, but also identifies the danger that such prescribing may inadvertently 'prolong the extent and frequency of continued injecting with the possibility of an increase in risk-laden behaviour'.

The prescription as the end state

It might be argued that there is not so much wrong with the end state of regular opiate use. Why is there such a preoccupation with habit-cessation? Although debaters have traditionally called upon evidence of damage associated with the opiates, it would appear that neuropsychological damage is only modest even after long-term injectable opiate use. The arguments seem to draw their lifeblood from moral or from organisational considerations. To what extent do we see the institutionalisation of the drug-taking behaviour as a legitimate form of treatment? In what way should we be gauging its effectiveness? Debate which straddles the Atlantic often fails to acknowledge the fundamentally different nature of some of the highly individual maintenance prescribing in the UK compared with its compartmentalised US equivalent. With the existence of injectable methadone maintenance within every UK doctor's armamentarium, the debate becomes more complicated and cannot be adequately dealt with by merely extrapolating the discussions that have taken place with regard to oral methadone maintenance.

It may be that oral methadone maintenance might come to be seen as an appropriate and acceptable intermediate goal if it was to be found that such oral maintenance reduced the extent of high-risk injecting and sexual activities; if so, then the organisational consequences are considerable and a large increase in the availability of places in prescribing programmes will be required, such as has been proposed in the report of US Presidential Commission on the Human Immunodeficiency Virus Epidemic (1988), which recommended the creation of 2,500 new treatment centres across the country and the appointment of 59,000 new staff so as to increase treatment availability to achieve 'treatment on demand'.

KEY ISSUES

Availability of less straightforward prescribing approaches

For some drug addicts, it may be appropriate to consider more unusual prescribing approaches – such as the prescribing of injectible methadone or injectible heroin in ampoule forms. It seems inappropriate for such complicated prescribing approaches to be implemented by doctors with less experience in the drug field, and so the ACMD (1988; 1989) have advocated a layered or stepped-care approach to prescribing, whereby more straightforward prescribing responses such as oral methadone withdrawals in the short and medium term should be available from general practitioners and district-level drug services, while more complicated prescribing responses such as possibly injectable methadone or heroin would require referral to more specialist drug units with more experienced staff and higher staff–patient ratios. As the treatment becomes more out of the ordinary, so the extent of safeguards for the service should become greater with the possible introduction of random urine analysis, home visits, telephone monitoring, and other such checks.

Availability of maintenance

With the benefit of hindsight, it is evident that the assurances of lifelong maintenance and consequent foreclosing of discussion about possible change would appear to have had some adverse effect on some of the long-term opiate addicts who have been with the NHS drug clinics in the UK since their creation in 1968. It is likely that approaches similar to those described above will be a more effective way of providing a service which is sensitive to the immediate needs of the individual while still promoting change in the drug-taking behaviour over time (see also Chapter 19). Thus, adoption of an end-state maintenance approach would be superseded by a more active approach which sought to identify a series of intermediate goals and looked at ways in which contingencies might be invoked and reinforcers identified so as to encourage appropriate changes in behaviour.

Availability of injectable drugs

Traditionally, this has been one of the special characteristics of prescribing in the UK. Even though any doctor may prescribe controlled drugs (including heroin and cocaine) to a patient for general medical purposes, it is only doctors with a special licence from the Home Office who may prescribe either heroin or cocaine to drug addicts in the treatment of their addiction. However, these specially licensed doctors (almost all of whom are in charge of drug dependence units) only rarely exercise this prescribing power. There remain many injectable forms of opiates which may be prescribed to a drug addict by any doctor in the UK and which are not covered by these special licensing requirements. In practice, the prescribing of injectable drugs is rare and is almost entirely restricted to injectable ampoules of methadone. The ACMD reports on *AIDS and Drug Misuse* (1988, 1989) explore the possible benefits that may result from the interim prescribing of injectable drugs as part of work towards an intermediate goal in carefully selected patients. The potential for serious error is greater in view of the much higher blackmarket value of these injectable drugs as well as more direct physical complications; and a careful cost–benefit analysis must be undertaken to examine the advantages and disadvantages of oral-only or part-injectable methadone prescription. However, in conducting such a cost–benefit analysis it is as well to include analysis of the likely outcome for prescribing other forms of methadone such as tablets; these are frequently crushed and injected, thereby exposing the drug user to a larger set of hazards than from injection of the prepared ampoules of methadone. The ever-present concern is that an injectable prescription might be given to a patient who could have been supported in making the move to an oral-only prescription but for whom the provision of a part-injectable prescription has confirmed the injecting behaviour.

The choice of drug on prescription is often the source of lively discussion, especially with commentators from outside the UK. Most attention is usually focused on whether or not heroin itself might be prescribed. However, in clinical practice a more critical issue is whether or not injectables are prescribed at all; the difference between injectable heroin and injectable methadone seems to be far less than the difference between injectable and/or oral forms of methadone, thus drawing attention to the importance that must be attached to the route of administration rather than merely the substance itself.

Prescribing stimulant drugs

It is interesting to consider why there is such a sharp distinction drawn between prescribing substitute drugs to opiate addicts and to amphetamine or cocaine addicts. While medium-term or long-term prescribing of methadone as a substitute opiate is commonly undertaken with heroin addicts, it is rare to find any consideration of similar prescribing of a stimulant substitute with the amphetamine or cocaine addict. Given the urgent need for there to be major changes in the injecting habits of many of these stimulant users, the possibility should at least be considered. However, in practice, it appears that all is not so straightforward, and certainly there is currently no candidate for occupying the role of a stimulant equivalent of methadone. The ACMD drew the conclusion from the limited evidence available that 'in practice, the prescription of stimulants is unlikely to lead to desirable changes in behaviour and carries a number of risks.' The only documented UK experiment into prescribing stimulant drugs to addicts was a short-lived experiment in the late 1960s which involved prescribing injectable methylamphetamine. The authors concluded that the experiment had been 'largely a record of therapeutic failure: it does not need a controlled trial to underline the fact that the help being given in our clinic was mostly ineffectual' (Mitcheson *et al.* 1976). Thus, despite the need to improve the 'capture' and 'retention' of stimulant users in the treatment service, it may well be necessary for us to look to non-pharmacological components which may fulfil these functions.

CONCLUSION

It is essential to understand that prescribing may occur within different contexts. A particular prescribing response may be life-saving or critical to a transition for one drug taker, while wholly inappropriate for the next. Any analysis of the range of necessary prescribing options must also consider which forms of prescribing should be available within which settings; it should also separately consider which forms of prescribing should exist within the total armamentarium of the overall service.

Occasionally debates about prescribing are productive and lead to an improved understanding on the part of the participants in the debate. However, more often the debate degenerates, producing more heat than light, with the debaters taking up well-rehearsed and repetitive points of view. At best, such debates are unproductive; at worst, they are actively damaging to the views of participants in the debate – and they certainly serve to drive away the partially interested audience who may happen to have dropped in on the debate. If we are to make any progress in our understanding of the range of possible prescribing interventions, we must avoid getting trapped into futile arguments in which there is a presumption that the prescribing question can be answered with a simple and universal 'yes' or 'no'.

REFERENCES

Advisory Council on the Misuse of Drugs (1988) *AIDS and Drug Misuse Report: Part I*, London: Department of Health.

Advisory Council on the Misuse of Drugs (1989) *AIDS and Drug Misuse Report: Part II*, London: Department of Health.

Gossop, M., Johns, A. and Green, L. (1986) 'Opiate withdrawal: in-patient versus out-patient programmes and preferred versus random assignment to treatment', *British Medical Journal* 293: 103–4.

Hartnoll, R.L., Mitcheson, M.C., Battersby, A., Brown, G., Ellis, M., Fleming, P. and Headley, N. (1980) 'Evaluation of heroin maintenance in controlled trial', *Archives of General Psychiatry* 37: 877–84.

Mitcheson, M., Edwards, G., Hawks, D. and Ogborne, A. (1976) 'Treatment of methylamphetamine users during the 1968 epidemic', in: G. Edwards, M.A.H. Russell, D. Hawks and M. MacCafferty (eds) *Drugs and Drug Dependence*, Farnborough: Saxon House/Lexington.

Presidential Commission on the Human Immunodeficiency Virus Epidemic (1988) *Report*, Washington.

Simpson, D.D. and Sells, S.B. (1983) 'Effectiveness of treatment for drug abuse: an overview of the DARP research program', *Advances in Alcohol and Substance Abuse* 2(1): 7–30.

Chapter Fourteen

THE ROLE OF HARM-REDUCTION PROGRAMMES IN CURBING THE SPREAD OF HIV BY DRUG INJECTORS

ERNST BUNING

In many countries the drug problem is approached with drug-free treatment programmes on the one hand, and law enforcement on the other. Generally this results in a limited number of drug takers in treatment and a marginalisation and criminalisation of drug users. Although this approach may be publicly attractive, it may be counterproductive in the long term.

To curb the spread of HIV within the drug-injecting population, and from them to the general population, it is essential to contact those drug users who are most at risk of becoming infected. Generally speaking, these individuals will avoid drug-free treatment programmes. Non-judgemental harm-reduction programmes may provide the best setting for HIV-prevention activities.

The Amsterdam experience shows that many drug users can be channelled through harm-reduction programmes to drug-free treatment and that these programmes are complementary rather than mutually exclusive. Although harm-reduction programmes may play a significant part in HIV prevention, in that they help to provide the necessary conditions for safer sex and safer drug use, there will always be those individuals who engage in risk-taking behaviour. This should not lead to defeatism. Our experience is that the majority of injecting drug users are willing to make behaviour changes, providing the conditions are right.

THE IDEA AND PRACTICE OF HARM REDUCTION

In most parts of the western world, treatment programmes actively pursue the goal of persuading drug users to abstain from the use of drugs. Although therapeutic treatment has greatly improved in the last two decades, success is limited; only a small percentage (10 to 20 per cent) of the drug-taking population is willing to enter therapeutic treatment. Of these, a stable drug-free life is accomplished by only 20 to 50 per cent (Sells and Simpson 1980). Abstinence-oriented programmes provide excellent services to those who are motivated to stop using drugs. The question remains as to what should be done about the remaining 80 to 90 per cent who are not. An answer to this question might be found by adopting a harm-reduction approach.

The rationale of harm reduction is: 'If it is not possible to cure drug users, one should at least try to minimise the harm that is being done both to them and the wider social environment.' The drug taker is helped through a difficult phase in life, whilst it is hoped, that in the longer term addiction may be overcome, either by treatment or natural recovery (Waldorf 1983). The effects of problem drug use, the spread of diseases and the problems for neighbourhoods caused by drug-related crime, are also targets of the harm-reduction philosophy.

In the development of an effective harm-reduction programme, the following questions must be considered: How can the programme contact as many drug users as possible? What measures are most effective in tackling the problem? What else can be done to motivate drug takers to enter treatment programmes and/or resocialisation projects? How can the burden on the broader society be minimised? These aspects will be illustrated by the experience of Amsterdam, where such programmes were initiated in 1981. This city, with about 7,000 hard-drug users (people who use heroin or cocaine), was one of the first places where pre-existing harm-reduction programmes were integrated into the HIV policy (Buning *et al.* 1988). While other countries may learn from the Amsterdam experience, every country will have to look for its own solutions that fit best with its culture.

REACHING AND CONTACTING DRUG USERS

For any harm-reduction programme to be effective it is essential to contact as many drug users as possible. In order to accomplish this, Amsterdam set up many outreach projects and established programmes that were attractive to drug takers. This included three special projects designed to contact those who would not actively seek help. First, streetworkers make frequent visits to places where concentrations of drug users can be found. They observe what is going on, provide verbal and/or written information and serve as a 'bridge' to helping institutions. The two foundations responsible for this streetwork employ about 30 streetworkers. Second, doctors from the Municipal Health Service visit local police stations twice a day to contact drug takers who have been arrested. Medical aid, including methadone, is administered, and as with the street-workers, the doctors provide information about existing help facilities. This project has proven to be most effective for all parties: withdrawal symptoms are treated; police work is freed from interruption by agitated suspects; and doctors gain first hand information of developments in the drug scene. Approximately 2,000 drug users are seen in the local police stations annually and 50 per cent have had no contact with a methadone programme in the year of their arrest. Third, a specialised team of social-psychiatric nurses visit the general hospitals. They counsel the drug takers who have been admitted and give advice to hospital staff. Their first priority is to facilitate general medical treatment. Once this is realised, possibilities for treating the patient's drug problem are considered. Approximately 350 patients are seen in the general hospitals each year.

THE AMSTERDAM HARM-REDUCTION PROGRAMMES

It is essential to provide help that is attractive to drug users and, furthermore, that the attitude of workers is non-judgemental. A moralistic approach is viewed as being counterproductive in that it would deter the majority of active drug users from seeking contact and help.

In Amsterdam, harm-reduction programmes operate at the primary care level and include social welfare and medical care. Drug users are given assistance with problems concerning housing, financial, and legal matters. This should not be regarded as 'maternalistic'; emphasis is placed on client responsibility, with social workers maintaining a friendly but firm attitude. Regular medical examinations are available, people can be referred to hospital, contraceptives are provided, needles and syringes can be exchanged, and methadone is distributed.

The role of methadone in harm reduction

Methadone distribution is considered a very powerful tool in attracting heroin users. Amsterdam has various methadone programmes. Annually, about 3,500 heroin addicts receive methadone from one of the facilities of the Municipal Health Service and approximately 50 per cent of the 400 general practitioners in Amsterdam prescribe methadone to about 1,500 patients. Since the Municipal Health Service refers patients to general practitioners and vice versa, there is some overlap between these two groups. Those working in the prescribing programmes, including general practitioners, are obliged to take part in a central methadone registration system. The most outreaching methadone programme is the low-threshold 'methadone bus' project. Every day two specially adapted city buses take a regular route through Amsterdam, stopping at a total of eight locations, each of which is in a drug-using area. In these buses liquid methadone is dispensed to heroin addicts who have been enrolled by and referred by one of the Municipal Health doctors. Participants are required to undergo a medical examination, but no urine test is necessary and there is no pressure to take part in counselling. The only conditions for participation are a means of identification (to prevent double prescribing), and a minimum contact with a medical practitioner of once every three months. No take-home dosages are issued and the single day's dose must be consumed under supervision. If patients repeatedly miss the bus they must return to the doctor. Nurses working on the methadone buses play a significant role in recognising people who suddenly deteriorate. In this project methadone is a means of contacting drug takers and provides a starting-point for the stabilisation of the patient's drug problem.

The methadone bus is a low-threshold programme. At the next level clients can be referred to one of three out-patient methadone clinics (*wijkposten*), on condition that they are willing to abstain from the use of illegal hard drugs such as heroin and cocaine. Here, urine checks are mandatory and counselling is provided. The advantage to the patient is that take-home dosages are allowed, for example, at weekends, and there is provision for counselling. Many patients of the *wijkposten* see their attendance as an improvement in their status over those who attend the methadone bus. As soon as a stable condition is achieved the client's general practitioner is asked to take over the methadone prescription.

Needle and syringe exchange

Needle and syringe exchange schemes are also attractive to active drug users who inject drugs. Of the estimated 7,000 problem drug users in Amsterdam, about 40 per cent inject (between 2,500 and 3,500). The remaining 60 per cent 'chase the dragon' (i.e. inhale the vapour of heated heroin) or inhale cocaine. The syringe-exchange schemes were initiated in the summer of 1984. This followed withdrawal of the daily sale of needles and syringes to about 200 addicts by a pharmacist in the inner-city area, which caused concern among workers in the field as well as drug injectors. Since an outbreak of hepatitis B was feared, the *junkiebond* (a league of drug addicts) proposed to start a needle and syringe exchange programme. Despite the initial fears of health authorities it was nevertheless decided that a small experiment within the *junkiebond* would be established. The Municipal Health Service bought a large stock of disposable needles and syringes, supplied them to the *junkiebond* at weekly intervals, and disposed of used ones. At the outset, approximately 1,000 needles and syringes were exchanged each week. When, during 1985, HIV became of growing concern, more institutions decided to participate in the exchange scheme (Buning *et al.* 1986). In 1986 the Municipal Health Service decided to make the exchange of needles and syringes available on the methadone buses as well. At 11 different locations injecting drug users can now exchange their used equipment for sterile needles and syringes. Between 1,500 and 1,750 users participate. In 1988 approximately 650,000 needles and syringes were exchanged. Findings from the first evaluation of the needle and syringe exchange (Hartgers *et al.* 1988) show that:

- i contact was made with injecting drug users who had no existing link with a methadone programme (25 per cent of the participants had not received methadone in the previous five years);
- ii no increase in drug use was reported amongst participants;
- iii participants in the exchange system showed less needle and syringe sharing than non-participants.

Information about HIV is given in both the methadone programmes and the needle and syringe exchange schemes. Personal contact (i.e. HIV counselling with attention for personal social skills) is considered to be the most effective means of persuading participants to practise both safer drug use and safer sex. However, information alone is not sufficient to curb the spread of HIV. Even if drug users have the social skills to get involved in safer behaviour, facilities have to be provided to make behaviour change possible; drug-free treatment for those who want to abstain, methadone for those who want to stop or reduce injecting and a needle and syringe exchange for those who want to avoid needle sharing. Condom slot machines were installed in all out-patient clinics and in the methadone buses, where the condoms can be obtained at a very low price; they are distributed free in a special VD clinic for prostitutes.

Harm reduction as part of a total helping system

We estimate that every year over 70 per cent of problem drug users are in touch with some part of the helping system. The Amsterdam experience has taught us that there is a place for both 'care' and 'cure'. The low-threshold methadone programme and the needle and syringe exchange schemes co-operate very effectively with drug-free therapeutic treatment programmes. They are complementary. Whilst clients are waiting to be admitted to a drug-free treatment clinic, they can make use of harm-reduction programmes. In this stage they are motivated to persevere with their decision. In practice, many clients are referred from harm-reduction programmes to drug-free treatment and resocialisation programmes. Since the introduction of harm-reduction programmes in 1981, the patient load of drug-free treatment and resocialisation programmes has more than doubled. During this period the total number of drug addicts has remained stable, and it appears that fewer young people have become heroin users.

The drug injector and the wider society

The assessment of harm-reduction programmes should not be limited simply to looking at the implications for individuals who are using drugs. Their behaviour has a major impact on society.

The Amsterdam programme works on the principle of reciprocity: goods and services are offered and in return clients are expected to behave in a socially acceptable manner. With the ready availability of methadone it is no longer necessary for drug users to become involved in drug-related crime which can be disruptive to others. Public health aspects should also be considered. A major concern is that HIV will spread from the drug-injecting population to the general population. The prevailing source of transmission will be through sexual contact. Addicted prostitutes are a particularly important potential source of transmission. It is self-evident that the sexual partner of the drug injector is as responsible for safer sexual practices as the drug injector. Nevertheless, the responsibility of the injector should also be stressed whenever HIV is being discussed in harm-reduction programmes. Another form of potential transmission of HIV to the general public is through needle-stick accidents. The most effective means of preventing this is to ensure that the number of contaminated needles in the environment is minimised. The needle and syringe exchange scheme provides an excellent means of collecting used needles and syringes.

PROBLEMS CONCERNING THE HARM-REDUCTION PROGRAMMES

The implementation of harm-reduction programmes is by no means a simple matter. There are considerable ideological issues to be considered. Not everyone is convinced of their value and there have been major debates between 'harm-reductionists' and workers in the drug-free treatment area. A number of individuals, some of whom have spent a lifetime in developing methods of curing addicts, regard them as a surrender to addiction. Many objections have been raised about syringe exchange as means of harm reduction. In Amsterdam, the objections are that:

i injecting drug abuse is encouraged and incentives to abstain are taken away;
ii people who inject drugs should be responsible for buying their own equipment;
iii needles and syringes from the exchange could be sold on the blackmarket to provide money for illegal drugs;

iv workers in the drug field are supposed to 'help', not to provide equipment that is harmful to individuals;
v pharmacists are discouraged from selling needles and syringes;
vi worker time could be spent on more meaningful and constructive activities.

It seems that workers in harm-reduction programmes have to prove themselves doubly. Most workers in such programmes will recognise the situation of having to answer questions from friends about the success rate of their programme: 'How many get off the drugs?' A difficult question if you are working in a needle and syringe programme.

In most harm-reduction programmes workers have to deal with the question of where to draw the line. Drug dealers and pushers may enter the facility and take over. Drug takers may try to sell stolen goods to personnel, and workers may be tempted to try hard drugs themselves. Rumours about the facility and negative press coverage may instil doubts in workers about the professional standard of their work. In this respect, it is of the utmost importance to be clear about the rules and regulations. Even a low-threshold facility should have boundaries, and these can be developed without creating a rigid and unfriendly climate.

The so-called 'burn-out' syndrome is another problem to be considered. Sooner or later many workers in harm-reduction programmes suffer from this. Having expended a great deal of energy upon improving the situation of drug users, they are all too often confronted with a relapse. With the introduction of HIV into the drug-injecting population the problem is exacerbated. The worker often feels powerless to influence the state of the client. To tackle this it is important to provide adequate staff training and to take denial and resistance among the staff seriously. Second, it is necessary to provide a long-term perspective for clients in terms of drug-free treatment and resocialisation.

The final problem is of a more political nature and concerns the 'international war on drugs'. Striving towards a drug-free society is a goal that is widely supported, especially those measures which are aimed at preventing problematic drug use. However, some of these may be counterproductive. If injecting drug users are driven underground, it will be almost impossible to reach them with information about safer sex and safer drug use. A climate of criminalisation and marginalisation is not conducive to positive behavioural changes. Politicians may have to decide which is the main priority, the fight against drugs or the fight against HIV.

REFERENCES

Buning, E.C., Coutinho, R.A. *et al.* (1986) 'Preventing AIDS in Amsterdam', *Lancet* i: 1435.

Buning, E.C., van Brussel, G.H.A. and van Santen, G. (1988) 'Amsterdam's drug policy and its implications for controlling needle sharing', in R.J. Battjes and R.W. Pickens (eds) *Needle Sharing among Intravenous Drug Abusers: National and International Perspectives*, Washington: National Institute on Drug Abuse, Research Monograph Series 80.

Hartgers, T., Buning, E.C. *et al.* (1988) 'Intraveneus druggebruik en het spuitenomruil programma in Amsterdam', *Tijdschrift Sociale Gezondheidszorg* 66: 207–10.

Sells, S.B. and Simpson, D.D. (1980) 'The case for drug abuse treatment effectiveness, based on the DARP research program', *British Journal of Addiction* 75(2): 117–31.

Waldorf, D. (1983) 'Natural recovery from opiate addiction: some social psychological processes of untreated recovery', *Journal of Drug Issues* 13(2): 237–80.

Chapter Fifteen

COMMUNICATIONS, EDUCATION, DRUGS AND HIV

NICHOLAS DORN AND NIGEL SOUTH

First the bad news. Education does not work as a means of prevention of illegal drug use. Nor do mass communications such as television commercials, street posters or newspaper announcements.

Yet since 1985, the British government has sponsored campaigns using print media, street posters, radio and television, focusing first on an anti-heroin message, then attempting to raise awareness of HIV in relation to sex, and by 1988 warning about the risks of injecting. Various styles have been used in these campaigns, including the abstract yet vaguely threatening imagery of the early 'iceberg' television commercials – there is more to an iceberg than you can see – which attempted to raise awareness about HIV; short cautionary tales in which man meets woman and an infection follows; illustrations of how HIV may be passed between people who share injection equipment; gruesome street posters picturing soiled and bloody syringes; and 'factual' style press advertisements signed by government chief medical officers. A few examples use humour, as in one television commercial in which a young man and woman exchange coy remarks about the last bus, before agreeing on safer sex. These anti-heroin, anti-injection and HIV campaigns have occurred in a context of increasing use of mass media by government to communicate on a variety of topics, including road safety, crime prevention, fire prevention, smoking and diet (see Anderson 1988, for a critique).

What can we say about the efficacy of these approaches? Our assertion that 'drug education does not work' rests on a firm basis of empirical evidence and sound theoretical considerations. At present the state of knowledge regarding the effectiveness of education in preventing behaviours encouraging the transmission of HIV is very limited. Examining drug education should be an instructive starting-point.

There are two broad kinds of reaction to the bad news that drug education does not work. The first is to take no notice and to carry on regardless, or (in a more sophisticated variation of carrying on regardless) to make tinkering changes of style, presentation and rationale. The second is to throw up one's hands in horror, and to say that if it doesn't work, then scrap it, and save the money. In part, the threat of this second reaction propels educators into a defence of the indefensible, and to a blocking of the possibilities for the more creative responses that come into view once we can see beyond the chimera of drug education/prevention.

In order to clear the ground towards a proper appraisal of the creative possibilities, it is useful to distinguish between two questions. First: 'What can education and mass media do for drug policy and practice?' Second: 'What can drug policy and practice do for education and the mass media?' How strange the second question sounds. We are so accustomed to seeing education and mass communications as *vehicles* for the traditional goal of reducing drug consumption, that it is hard to conceive of a situation in which drug-related activities might *contribute* to the specific purposes of the school curriculum, to the practice of social education in the youth service, to the goals of community education, or to the aims of local radio or national entertainment programmes. Such considerations may seem shallow compared with the urgency of 'the war against drugs', and it may be unexpected to find these issues raised in a book dedicated to an understanding of issues around drugs and HIV. But there lies the problem – the implicit assumption that any context, any curriculum, any channel of communication can and should be bent to the purposes of drugs/HIV education. What follows questions this assumption.

OVERVIEW OF THE EVALUATION EVIDENCE

It is sometimes said that as yet there is insufficient evidence of the effectiveness, ineffectiveness or side-effects of drug education. This is not really true. There is a quite considerable English-language literature on evaluations of drug education in schools and colleges, covering up to 200 drug education programmes. The general conclusion to be drawn from the more scientifically conducted studies – which use experimental and control groups, measures of self-reported behaviour change over several months, and some monitoring of the actual delivery of the educational programme – is that no known kind of drug education is capable of reducing experimentation with illegal drugs (Casswell *et al.* 1982; De Haes 1988; Schaps *et al.* 1988). Whether the approach uses fear, facts, de-emphasises substances in order to focus upon people and values, or looks at choice-situations and decision-making skills, drug education does not decrease the rate of experimentation.

One of the features of drug education internationally is for rapid changes in fashion, and for each new approach to be hailed as the answer until the evaluation evidence is produced. The middle to late 1980s was a propitious time for 'Just Say No' approaches, just as in earlier years fear approaches 'balanced' factual approaches and person-focused approaches played on the claimed efficacy of their own educational styles. Evaluators have dealt such claims some uncomfortable knocks. Their refrain – you can increase knowledge, shift attitudes, but you cannot change behaviour – seems likely to continue to be applicable in drug education, health education, and their variants in schools, colleges and other institutional settings.

When it comes to mass communications, such as television commercials or press advertisements, the situation seems somewhat similar. The British situation provides an interesting case because, following a high-level policy decision to proceed with campaigns on heroin, drugs and HIV, and sexuality and HIV, evaluation evidence relating to these campaigns is now available. First, there are studies using qualitative methods of group discussion and/or in-depth interviews, focusing upon questions of if and how to mount particular campaigns (Andrew Irving Associates 1985). Second, there are quantitative studies repeated at several points in time, intended to reveal evidence of the effectiveness of the first wave of advertising, which was anti-heroin in its focus and message (Research Bureau Ltd 1986). Third, there are evaluations that draw upon qualitative and quantitative evidence to paint a more general picture of the reception (by the general population and social groups therein) of HIV-related campaigns (Department of Health and Social Security and Welsh Office 1987). The findings of these latest evaluations are compatible with those of institutional educational programmes, but contribute some observations about specific social groups. Broadly speaking:

i Some specific population groups (of which the clearest example is the gay community) were *ahead* of the campaigns; indeed, were influences upon the campaigns (rather than vice versa). In these cases the campaigns may have reinforced changes that were already occurring.

ii Other population groups – in particular, drug injectors not in touch with treatment agencies or other drug services – have a relatively low awareness of anti-injection campaigns and the majority seem to be continuing to share injection equipment and engaging in unsafe sex.

iii General population groups (e.g. parents and most young people) fall between concerned gays and promiscuous syringe sharers in their responses. There is a tendency for these groups to call for more 'realism' (for which read 'strong' messages) in relation to drugs, and to display an ambiguous attitude to the issue of safer sex ('important, but not for me').

These general findings bring out the importance of the culture of social groups. Male gay culture has a self-confessed history of promiscuity – but that history has been thrown into sharp relief by the strength of the struggle to save lives and rebuild the community in a more settled and caring form. Male gay culture has specific strengths upon which it has successfully drawn to meet a mortal challenge and to push back anti-gay prejudice. Contrast this with the cultures surrounding unsafe injection in the hidden sector of drug injectors. It is not that such groups lack a culture; on the contrary, the cultures of needle-sharing groups may often be very strong, and strong in ways that render current HIV advertisements ineffective.

CONSUMING COMMUNICATIONS: LOOKISM AND DESIGNER HEALTH PROMOTION

A message that does not resonate – in the culture of those who receive it – with the meanings intended by those who designed it is a useless (and potentially harmful) message. In order to assess what might be a useful message, one has to start with an examination of the culture(s) in which one hopes to resonate. When this essential stage is missed out the prospects for effective communications are low.

Let us explore this by discussing an aspect of male gay cultures and contrasting this with cultures of drug injectors. We use the term 'lookism' to refer to an aspect of culture in which looking at self and others provides a basis for interaction between people and for evaluation of oneself and other people. There are two broad forms of lookism: the 'nice' variety (for example, looking young, healthy, beautiful and sexy); and the self-consciously 'nasty' variety (for example, presenting oneself as rough and/or as damaged by society). Nice, narcissistic lookism is an attribute of some male gay cultures in the main metropolitan centres in western nations in which a definable and public gay culture has emerged. Contrast this with the cultures of many groups of drug injectors. Here, there is no investment in looking healthy. Indeed, looking and acting a bit 'wrecked' is more attractive. This 'nasty' version of lookism means that any strategy that stands on 'nice' lookist assumptions (such as parts of the British government campaigns) would be wrongly positioned as far as many injectors are concerned. In a culture where damage to appearance and to health is worn with pride, health education exhortations warning of physical ill-health and incapacitation are hardly likely to have preventive impact.

Let us now look at the interactions that occur around drink and drugs in some subcultures of drug injectors. Commentators have linked the problem of needle sharing with the issue of 'trust'. The idea is that there is no greater insult than to refuse to share food, drink and other things with one's friends: refusal may be taken as evidence that one is an enemy rather than a friend; and pressures to share are especially strong between close friends, sexual partners or others who regard themselves as bound by specific emotional ties and broader cultural orientations. 'Why won't you share with me – do you not trust me?' is a powerfully disciplinary form of words. It is not so much that there is a generalised 'problem of sharing', but rather that a mixture of inattention to and celebration of bodily risks and physical disfigurement is part of the cultures of various depressed social groups. Some alternative to traditional health education is clearly needed in these circumstances and other approaches are discussed in Dorn (1989), Gamble and Fraser (1988), Gilman (1988) and Newcombe (1988).

PRODUCING COMMUNICATIONS: HOW PARTICULAR MEDIA, CONTEXTS AND COMMITMENTS SHAPE MESSAGES

Communications can be produced in a variety of media. What may be a suitable message in one of these media may sit strangely in another. It comes as no surprise, then, that advertising agencies vary the style and content of advertisements according to the medium being used. Those used in the 'youth press' differ from those of television commercials not only in the obvious sense that the first are based around still images whilst the second use moving pictures: the printed adverts also present an image reflecting a particular slice of time, whilst film media encourage the portrayal of an interaction, process or history, in one or more vignettes. During late 1988, anti-HIV adverts intended for drug takers tended to be presented in the form of street posters, whilst anti-HIV commercials intended for heterosexuals tended to be presented in the form of television commercials. The print and poster presentation of anti-sharing messages pushed them away from 'human interest' (which thrives on process, interaction, story-telling) and towards 'impact' (needles, bloody cloth, etc.). The filmed and processual nature of television, on the other hand, positively encourages story-telling on the basis of close observation of one or more characters. British television commercials encouraging the use of condoms by heterosexuals positively invite the viewer to identify with the build-up to a sexual encounter, and the nemesis that follows. Contrast this successful use of the medium with the very first anti-HIV commercials on British television, in which some combination of haste and uncertainty amongst the sponsors and producers of the commercial resulted in an attempt to portray a primarily static image – icebergs. This commercial reportedly provoked much audience confusion, and subsequent campaigns have used print and television media more appropriately.

Another context in which there is a close relation between the media and the message is the school. Here we can identify three distinct approaches to drug/HIV education. Proponents of the first approach – whom we could call the Traditionalists – say that, in so far as there is explicit discussion about these difficult issues in schools, a strong moral line must form the framework for specific bits of information or advice. A group that we call the Subject Educators argue that the school is an institution that instils competence in particular ways of thinking (e.g. mathematical thinking) and that issues such as sex, drug use, infection and health should be dealt with within *every* subject in ways appropriate to that subject. (This most closely corresponds to the authors' own position.) Third, there is a large but declining group, which we call the Progressives, who advocate a social-psychological approach to discovery and cultivation of self by small group techniques focusing upon self-esteem and decision-making skills, calling for more space in the school curriculum for these approaches under such titles as personal, social and health education.

What stands between these positions is *not* a difference of view about the efficacy of their versions of education as drug prevention. There is little debate about effectiveness. What is at stake is the broader question of what a school is or should be. Is it, as the Traditionalists would have it, a cross between the patriarchal family, the factory and the army? If so, then 'moral instruction' is in order. Is it, as the Progressives would say, a free and nurturing space within which the self is cultivated? If so, then personal, social and health education of a psychologically inclined kind is in order. Or is a school, as Subject Educators claim, a place where young people develop the ability to think about the world from a variety of vantage-points and become competent in a number of spoken and written discourses, based on subject learning? If so, then subject-based drugs/sex education across the whole curriculum is appropriate. We believe that this last approach most closely corresponds to the concept of schooling in popular cultures (ethnic and religious minority cultures included), and is the framework of orientation within which most students (and teachers) engage. Fitting into this framework of expectations seems more appropriate than not doing so.

In this section we have discussed some ways in which both the context of the communication, and producers' ideas about the right use of those contexts shape the kinds of messages that can be given. The general conclusion to be drawn is that communication contexts vary quite markedly between themselves and so do producers' commitments to how to work within each of these contexts. It follows that no single or uniform message can be given across all channels of communication. The analysis in this chapter points towards a position of pluralism in drugs/HIV education, where the different presentations are shaped to take into consideration the contexts in which messages are produced (the opportunities and constraints of television, print media, school curricula, etc.), and the contexts in which they are consumed (i.e. the cultures of specific social groups).

TOWARDS A FRAMEWORK OF ACTION

So far, if only by default, the emphasis has implicitly fallen upon the first question outlined in the introduction – what can education and the mass media do for drug/HIV policy and practice? Let us now try to pull together two dimensions of our argument:

- i the distinction between a focus on consumers, and a focus on producers of communications; and
- ii the distinction between communications as a tool of HIV policy, and HIV presentations as supporting particular interests of communications and educational specialists.

These two dimensions are put together in Table 15.1. Most discussions of education/communications and HIV have assumed that communications work or can be made to work in the service of HIV policy. Also, the focus has been more upon the person consuming the message, than upon its producers. These assumptions describe a well-known model in mass communications and educational circles – the Effects Model. This model underlies research that examines the 'impact' or 'effects' of messages on individuals to see, for example, if they adopt safer sexual or drug-using practices in response to exposure to particular messages.

Part of the difficulty with the Effects Model is highlighted by the so-called Uses and Gratifications Model. This emphasises the extent to which the existing characteristics of individuals, small groups and cultures can selectively perceive messages or parts of messages, can rework themes to make sense to the individual and the small groups within which the issues are discussed, and can result in messages being taken up in ways that interest and gratify viewers/readers (but may never have been envisaged by the people who produced the message). From this point of view, one should be starting with an examination of the culture of a social group, and trying to build a message on top of the existing perceptions and interests of the group.

Table 15.1 Four models of communications about HIV

	Focus on consumers of communications	*Focus on producers of communications*
Communications in the service of HIV policy	Effects Model – communications change views and behaviour of those who consume them.	Agenda-setting Model – producers of communications make HIV an issue for other producers.
HIV policy in the service of existing interests	Uses and Gratifications Model – consumers of communications use them selectively to bolster existing views.	Market Share Model – producers of communications rework HIV issues to fit into their existing commitments.

Turning now to communications in relation to those who produce them, the well-known Agenda-setting Model describes a situation in which media define the public agenda – crime, economic matters, health – and define the issues on the agenda (for example, as street crime, strikes, infection spread by outsiders, etc.). In the Agenda-setting Model communications enterprises borrow popular themes from each other and build up a shared definition of the issues of the day. The emphasis is upon the ways in which communicators influence each other into reproducing a certain issue as part of the public agenda. Every day newspaper staff review last night's television, and every day television researchers and producers read the papers, to see what has and what has not been defined as an issue by others. One tends, therefore, to get 'waves' of reporting – solvents, heroin, cocaine, AIDS, Ecstasy, etc. Similar and related waves occur in educational systems, as key persons react to wider issues culled from the mass media.

Lastly, the Market Share Model focuses upon competition between agencies that produce mass communications and educational products and services. Such competition takes two broad and related forms: competition over ideological and frankly political matters (e.g. the characteristics of a nation, leadership, public morality, 'folk devils', etc.) and over sales volumes and profitability of products and services. News organisations, entertainment enterprises, health promotion agencies, educational institutions and self-help groups struggle to win the political argument and to retain or increase economic viability, and in practice success on one front is linked to success on the other. We think that this model of understanding HIV-related communications and education – as aspects of competitive relations between ideologically literate and cash-hungry agencies – helps to pinpoint the basic realities in the field. When one hears it said of a communications or educational agency that 'they've done well', this is not necessarily understood solely as a reference to saving people from HIV. The reference is equally likely to be to the increased stature and budget of the agency concerned.

The problem with a multiplicity of models is that, since each model directs attention to some aspects of a phenomenon but not to others, one ends up confused. This is a fruitful state to be in, as long as the experience is temporary. In moving towards our conclusion, therefore, we want to suggest a procedure by which people planning or reviewing communications or education in the area of drugs/HIV may highlight four key questions by going through each of the models in a particular order:

- i What broad ideological commitments and economic targets of our agency have to be satisfied by any intervention we might make? (Market Share Model of communications as competition.)
- ii What do we know about the cultures of the social groups with whom we are trying to communicate, such that we can identify existing ideas that have currency in the culture, and can build upon them? (Uses and Gratifications Model.)
- iii Can we devise ways of making a particular message (derived from a study of the social group, step (ii) above) be taken up by other news and educational agencies, who accept it as an important public issue? If so, then we multiply our messages for free, and reach further than by relying on our own messages alone. (Agenda-setting Model.)
- iv Lastly, to what extent are the messages perceived, attended to,

discussed or acted upon by the groups for whom they were intended? (Effects Model, employed as part of an evaluation.)

We offer these four questions as a realistic structure for agencies in approaching action in the fields of communications, education, drugs and HIV.

CONCLUSION

The proper roles of education and mass communications in relation to HIV and drugs are a matter for continuing debate. Education can raise issues, set agendas, and is likely to be taken up selectively by different social groups – but no single message or medium has the power to effect a general transformation of behaviour across all social groups. Therefore, educators and communicators have to be modest and pragmatic. We have offered a framework – moving through four key questions – that may be useful for those wishing to develop or evaluate HIV/drugs education. Educators and communicators need to be clear about their own commitments and those of their organisation, to assess the qualities of the medium or educational setting in which they are working, to assess the chances that their message will be 'newsworthy' in the eyes of other organisations, and to take on board the concerns and cultures of the people they wish to address.

REFERENCES

Anderson, D. (1988) *The Megaphone Solution*, London: Social Affairs Unit.

Andrew Irving Associates (1985) *Heroin Misuse Publicity Campaign: A Qualitative Study Designed to Guide the Effective Targetting and Development of a Mass Media Campaign*, London: Andrew Irving Associates.

Casswell, S., Mortimer, D. and Gilroy, C. (1982) 'The minimal effects and methodological problems in the evaluation of a harm-reduction drug education programme in a high school setting', *Journal of Drug Education* 12(4): 345–52.

De Haes, W. (1988) 'Drug education? Yes, but how?', *Addictive Behaviours*, Edinburgh: Scottish Health Education Group.

Department of Health and Social Security and Welsh Office (1987) *AIDS Monitoring Response to the Public Education Campaign*, February, 1986–February, 1987, London: HMSO.

Dorn, N., (1989) 'British policy on prevention', in A. Ghodse and C. Kaplan (eds) *Responding to Drug Problems: An Anglo-Dutch Debate,* Parthenon Publishing.

Gamble, L. and Fraser, R. (1988) 'Local radio as a strategy in reducing drug related harm', in N. Dorn, L. Lucas and N. South (eds) *Drug Questions 4,* London: Institute for the Study of Drug Dependence.

Gilman, M. (1988) 'Comics as a strategy in reducing drug-related harm', in: N. Dorn, L. Lucas and N. South (eds) *Drug Questions 4,* London: Institute for the Study of Drug Dependence.

Newcombe, R. (1988) 'Serious fun: drug education through popular culture', *Druglink* 3(6): 11–13.

Research Bureau Ltd (1986) *Report of Findings: Stages I-III,* London: Research Bureau Ltd.

Schaps, E., Di Bartolo, R., Palley, C. and Churgin, S. (1981) 'A review of 127 drug abuse prevention programmes', *Journal of Drug Issues* 11(1): 17–43.

Chapter Sixteen

REACHING OUT TO INJECTING DRUG USERS

SAMUEL R. FRIEDMAN, CLAIRE STERK, MERYL SUFIAN, DON C. DES JARLAIS AND BRUCE STEPHERSON

Outreach to injecting drug users around AIDS risk reduction has been developed most extensively in the United States. It was started in a few areas such as New Jersey, New York City, and San Francisco, and has since become the focus of a large-scale, multiple-city national initiative by the National Institute on Drug Abuse. The US focus on outreach is probably a result of four facts that together push the USA towards outreach as a way to produce risk reduction. First, the AIDS epidemic among injecting drug users developed first and hardest in the New York City region. Second, most injecting drug users in the USA are not in regular communication with drug treatment services or other social agencies, so any attempt to provide them with information has to set up new channels of communication. Third, political and other pressures in the USA have delayed or prevented the establishment of syringe exchanges or even of adequate drug treatment capacity, so preventing the spread of HIV has had to rely on messages or on distributing bleach and condoms rather than on providing injectors with the means for self-protection. Fourth, both the high salience of individualistic belief systems and the concomitant existence of a long tradition of health education predispose public health officials to act primarily in terms of providing messages about individual behaviour change rather than organising collective risk reduction and campaigns.

The goal of most outreach has been to provide injecting drug users and their sexual partners with information about how to protect themselves. At its minimum, this involves information about how HIV is transmitted and about what behaviours need to be altered to protect oneself or to keep from transmitting HIV to others if one is already infected. The goal of such communication is usually conceptualised as being behaviour change. Many outreach projects in the USA have distributed condoms and bleach, as well as messages, to injecting drug users. (Bleach is used to decontaminate syringes. It has been demonstrated that it does this for free HIV and also that it inactivates infected white blood cells so that proviral HIV that has been integrated into cell DNA is unable to produce more HIV (Keddie *et al.* 1988).) Distributing bleach and condoms not only provides drug users with the means for reducing risks, but also is a powerful means of communicating the actuality of risk reduction by dramatising both the need for protection and the mechanisms through which it can be accomplished.

More sophisticated formulations understand that risk behaviours occur within social relationships, and thus also provide messages and other assistance to help users and partners transform relationships in ways that enable risk reduction to occur. Some of these relationships are dyads or small groups. Examples include friendship groups who shoot up together and pairs of drug users who are involved in steady sexual relationships. The need to consider relationships rather than just behaviours is clarified by considering that beginning to use condoms can threaten the survival of a sexual partnership and all the emotional and economic benefits that are derived from it. One study found that the sexual relationships of a number of seropositive men ended when they tried to protect their partners (Casadonte *et al.* 1986). On the other hand, interventions with injecting drug users need to take into account the looseness and predatory aspects of many of their social relationships (Des Jarlais *et al.* 1986).

As will be discussed later, wider subcultural and societal social relationships provide a context for risk behaviours that occur within small group relationships. One form of outreach tries to organise drug users and/or partners to push for small group, subcultural, and perhaps even societal changes that will facilitate risk reduction. These attempts to produce subcultural change tend to be more complex. The logic is that subcultural change goes beyond the individual, and tries to enlist peer pressure as a force for risk reduction.

All these efforts are shaped by the nature of social relationships and networks among injecting drug users in an area; by their relationships with official society and with people in general; and different kinds of outreach or community intervention may be more or less successful at reaching different kinds of users.

INDIVIDUALLY FOCUSED INTERVENTIONS

New Jersey has been in a unique position in the United States since injecting drug users have comprised the majority of its AIDS cases. This helped concentrate public health attention on drugs and AIDS, and led to New Jersey setting up the first AIDS outreach project for drug users. These outreach efforts began in 1985 when the state drug agency funded drug treatment centres to hire ex-addict outreach workers. Their initial focus was on communicating techniques for safer injection to drug users, and they specifically decided not to use the outreach workers to recruit users into drug abuse treatment. None the less, they found that many of the injecting drug users to whom outreach workers spoke applied for treatment (Jackson and Rotkiewitz 1987). They then began having outreach workers distribute coupons that allowed the recipients to receive free drug detoxification services. (New Jersey had instituted charges for detoxification after the federal budget cuts of the early 1980s; these charges meant that many users felt priced out of the market for drug detoxification just as AIDS began to appear.) More recently, outreach workers have co-ordinated their efforts with mobile health vans which take teams of medical service providers and counsellors into areas where drug users congregate or where the sex partners of drug users are likely to be found. These teams provide a wide range of services, including referrals to treatment, medical examinations and HIV antibody tests (along with pre-test and post-test counselling).

The San Francisco outreach project was developed on the basis of years of prior ethnographic study of the drug scene. Harvey Feldman, Patrick Biernacki and John Newmeyer reasoned that injectors were too busy to make major changes in their drug-taking patterns; thus, any risk-reduction technique would have to be easily incorporated into their routines or it would not be implemented. They decided that cleaning injection equipment with bleach and then rinsing it with fresh water would be a feasible and effective method of decontaminating the equipment. They then devised an outreach scheme that would let them spread this message to the user community. They did this by hiring streetwise, committed outreach workers who were not ex-users, and training them in how to interpret events on the street and how to communicate effectively with drug users. These outreach workers then were sent into the streets with bottles of bleach and with condoms and literature. Reports by Watters (1987) and Moss and Chaisson (1988) suggest that a large percentage of injectors in San Francisco have begun regularly to clean their equipment with bleach.

Even though New York City studies had indicated that most injectors knew about the basic routes of HIV transmission, the New York City AIDS Outreach Project was originally established with educational aims. It planned to reinforce lessons users already knew, to reach the minority who had not yet learned these basics, to counteract dangerously false rumours, and to inform drug users about risk-reducing behavioural strategies and negotiating techniques with groups of drug users (Friedman *et al.* 1986).

Teams of ex-addict educators were sent into the streets to tell injectors about the dangers of AIDS and about risk-reduction strategies. The outreach effort offered the users the opportunity to receive antibody testing and the associated pre- and post-test counselling, and assisted interested users to enter drug treatment programmes. Substantial programme drift occurred, however, in that more outreach worker effort focused on getting users and their sexual partners to come in for antibody testing than had been anticipated. Relatively little educational effort was observed by the project's ethnographer, and only a minority of subjects who answered a questionnaire when they came in to be tested reported that the outreach workers had taught them about HIV transmission routes. In spite of this programme drift, however, preliminary analysis of 144 subjects who came in to be tested (and thus received counselling at the test site), and who were able to be re-interviewed three to 11 months later, suggests that the project had a salutary effect on levels of risk behaviour. Thus, drug injection frequency, the proportion of injections which occurred in shooting galleries, the frequency of sex without condoms, and the proportion of sexual encounters in which male drug users had unprotected sex, all decreased.

SUBCULTURAL CHANGE

In Chicago, an outreach project that had its roots in the theory underlying the San Francisco project and in many years of ethnographic work among local users went one step further in conceiving how to produce risk reduction. Wayne Wiebel developed ideas of intervention that involved hiring locally influential drug users to distribute information, bleach and condoms to local users in their friendship groups and to the friends of their friends. Underlying this was a model of subcultural permeation that may be more appropriate in Chicago than in New York or some other cities. Persons with influence among drug users – whom we might describe as 'sociometric stars' – could easily reach out to large numbers of users (and their sexual partners) through their friendship networks, and these networks would utilise the influential personalities' prestige to change the norms, values and practices of the local user community. Supervision of the project was vested in ethnographers who ran each field station; these ethnographers were in charge of locating the influential people, hiring them, showing them how to do outreach and discharging them when and if they exhausted their usefulness to the project. In the period during which the project has been in operation, this model has succeeded in attracting several thousand users for risk assessments and interview.

Some HIV outreach efforts, including some of the most innovative attempts to help the drug user subculture change in ways that facilitate risk reduction, have been established by drug users on their own behalf. Prior to the discovery of AIDS, drug users in the Netherlands had formed organisations to defend their dignity and to press for changes in drug treatment policies and police practices (see Chapter 14; Friedman and Casriel 1988; Friedman *et al.* 1987). The Rotterdam *junkiebond* set up a needle-exchange programme, including sporadic street distribution to prostitutes, in response to a hepatitis B epidemic in the early 1980s. This was expanded, with financial assistance from public health authorities, when AIDS became a visible threat. The Rotterdam *junkiebond* produced a pamphlet that described the risks and that recommended ways in which drug users could reduce their risk. Later, these anti-AIDS efforts spread to other *junkiebonden* and to the Netherlands Federation of *Junkiebonden* (FNJB). Indeed, the secretariat of the FNJB has been actively involved in going to local users' groups and getting them involved in making educational videos about AIDS – which has been an effective way to get users committed to AIDS education and risk-reduction efforts directed at other users.

Unlike gays, injecting drug users in the USA have not established collective organisations of their own. This has prevented them from developing a consciously directed sense of solidarity and of self-defence against HIV, and has probably retarded risk reduction (Friedman *et al.* 1987). In an effort to determine whether drug users' organisations can be initiated by outside organisers, and whether such externally instigated organisations can mount effective risk-reduction campaigns, we (together with ADAPT, an organisation of ex-users and health professionals dedicated to stopping the spread of HIV and to ameliorating its effects) have been engaged in an organising campaign in the Williamsburg section of Brooklyn (see Friedman and Casriel (1988) for a discussion of some of the differences between outside organising and spontaneous self-organisation of drug users). Initial trust was gained by having ADAPT hire ex-addict organisers to work intensively with the users in a limited section of Williamsburg. The organisers distributed bleach, condoms and other risk-reduction materials; educated users about AIDS; helped sick users get hospital care and drug treatment; helped users in other ways, particularly in relation to getting social services; and generally acted as friends who recognised the human worth and dignity of the users they came to know. One effort to build solidarity and reduce the risk of accidental HIV transmission involved organising the residents and *habitués* of one abandoned building (the site of a number of shooting galleries) to remove used syringes, garbage, and debris from the area. More than 30 meetings have been held with the female injecting drug prostitutes in this area, and meetings of male drug users have started. Although it is too early to determine whether these efforts have led to large-scale risk reduction, and although the organisations are still nascent rather than clear successes, we would argue that the degree of organisation that has been reached is greater than many would have thought possible. Further organising, and research to evaluate the effects of this organising on risk behaviour and on social relationships that affect risk behaviour, are being conducted.

OUTREACH AS WORK

It is important not to view outreach only in terms of its stated goals. Outreach is a form of human activity, and thus its implementation depends upon the efforts of outreach workers. These outreach workers are usually employees of one or another community or government agency. As such, they are subject to the social dynamics that are usually analysed in the sociology of work. Further, the social relations of their work – both in terms of their relationship to their employer and colleagues, and in terms of how their tasks define their relationships to injectors or other community residents – can have considerable impact on what occurs and what can be attempted in a given community.

Our discussion of outreach as work is based on ethnographic observation of projects in several cities and on conversations with outreach workers or research staff from other projects. The remarks in this section, then, should not be interpreted as definitive, but rather as suggesting ideas for future research.

Usually, ex-users are hired as outreach workers because they know the ins and outs of the subculture, including its language and values, and are thus able to communicate, win trust, and/or organise effectively. A major reason why some projects avoid hiring ex-users is that they fear ex-users will be unable to resist the temptation to inject once they are exposed to active drug users and see drugs being used in the course of their work. Indeed, although studies have not been done to estimate the extent of such relapse – and have also not compared the extent of relapse to that which might have been expected in the absence of being given jobs as outreach workers – there have been a considerable number of cases of relapse among outreach workers in the USA.

Projects differ in what they mean by an 'ex-addict outreach worker'. Some projects that want outreach workers who can most thoroughly blend in with the user community are relatively lax about rules concerning drug use. For instance, one pattern is for the employer to demand that the outreach workers do not get high when on the job or in public. Other projects want to be sure their outreach workers do not use drugs other than their prescribed supply; these projects usually seek workers with more time in treatment and, perhaps, with more education.

Since the way in which the employment relationship is

organised can affect the delivery of services, it is useful to consider the benefits and problems of work as an outreach worker. First, consider pay. Many ex-user outreach workers are hired from among the unemployed or from low-paying, part-time service or human service jobs. This reflects the fact that the job prospects of ex-users are not good (indeed, many of them may have become users because of the dismal economic prospects for youth raised in their neighbourhoods). Other outreach workers are hired from jobs in drug treatment agencies, where they may have had responsible positions, because they want to be more directly involved in stopping the spread of HIV.

Outreach workers seem often to be hired at rates of pay that are reasonably high for their neighbourhoods – but relatively low for the cities in which they live. In New York City annual full-time pay levels for different projects have ranged between $14,000 and $20,000 for outreach *per se* during 1988. Many outreach workers, however, have been given only half-time work. Outreach workers often express a desire to have a career ladder which would offer hope for an improved standard of living and for recognition of their contributions. A career ladder also validates their self-esteem, since it means that they are considered capable of helping to plan and direct projects of this importance. In the absence of such career ladders, staff turnover is quite high, and few outreach workers stay on the job as long as two years. In the New York City project only seven of the first 20 outreach workers remain employed after about two years, and all of these have received promotions to supervisory field positions of one kind or another.

Projects attempt to give outreach workers non-monetary rewards to supplement their pay. On the one hand, this is easy – outreach work, when successful, has a clear social utility that saves the lives of people with whom the worker associates. Further, some prestige may accrue to the worker from being part of an organisation that often includes scientists or agency directors who receive considerable publicity for what they are doing about AIDS. More concretely, drug users frequently express their gratitude to outreach workers for what they are doing. For ex-user outreach workers, who often grew up with little expectation of ever working in a job that would involve such appreciation and utility, these rewards can be a powerful motivating factor.

It is, however, important to understand the limits of these

non-monetary rewards in motivating outreach workers. The benefits of working at a life-saving occupation are eroded by the daily realities of working in dangerous, grimy, drug settings and by the diseases and other problems that they see drug users falling prey to. Furthermore, to the extent that users try to manipulate their relationships to outreach workers (and this is frequent), cynicism sets in. Also, the rewards of working with high-prestige professionals can easily vanish, or even turn into bitterness, if outreach workers feel that they are not treated with dignity and respect. We hypothesise that rigid labour control systems that are sometimes set up to prevent the relapse of ex-user outreach workers may sometimes implicitly convey a message that management does not trust the workers. If so, this may detract from the willingness of outreach workers to put forward their best efforts. It is also our tentative observation that projects in which outreach workers have little autonomy are more likely to experience low morale than are projects where outreach workers have autonomy and initiative.

The way in which outreach workers relate to local users can affect how they feel about their jobs. Projects in which the outreach workers are recruited from and remain within a given neighbourhood, or where they work intensively to become part of the neighbourhood scene over a period of months, can produce positive social relationships between project staff and local users (and other residents), and this produces high morale and a willingness to make extra efforts to help those in need. On the other hand, it is more likely that there will be low morale among outreach workers on projects in which the workers' task is defined primarily in terms of getting a message out to the users quickly, and then moving on to the next neighbourhood, or in which outreach workers are assigned to recruit people to take part in counselling or other activities in another area.

In some projects in the USA, also, there has been racial tension either between some of the outreach workers and some of the local users or between some outreach workers and project management. We would hypothesise that this is particularly likely in areas where the users are of various races and feel a degree of hostility or fear towards users of other races.

Although we initially believed that outreach workers would usually be most effective with injectors of their own gender, our ethnographic observations suggest that this may not always be the case. In at least two settings that we have observed, it appears that male outreach workers are most effective in communicating with female users, and the female outreach workers with male users. On the other hand, for more intense outreach work that goes beyond simple communication to deal with intimate personal issues or for some parts of organising efforts, it appears that the most effective work is done by outreach workers or organisers of the same gender as the user(s) being worked with.

In concluding this section, we want to re-emphasise an earlier point. These observations about outreach as work are meant to encourage systematic research and to serve as a source of hypotheses for future testing.

CONCLUSION

In considering the experience of outreach work so far, we are impressed by the extent to which projects have been willing to experiment with ideas that conventional wisdom would have questioned. For example, many drug treatment agencies have recognised the need to work with users on issues other than getting them to enter treatment; in many cases, they have then been gratified to find that such efforts produce a widespread desire to enter treatment and quit using drugs.

Many factors may affect the success or failure of a given outreach approach in a particular city. The social welfare laws, drug policies and racial and ethnic structures of the Netherlands may explain why drug users there have formed associations whereas this has not occurred in the USA. The extent to which injecting drug users have fixed residences and are part of stable neighbourhood friendship or kinship networks may determine whether the Chicago networking model can be applied. Comparative research on a multi-city or international basis can help us understand what factors have such effects, and thus can indicate what approaches may work in a given city or with a given subpopulation of drug users. Implementation of outreach projects has relied primarily on ethnographic and drug treatment practitioners' knowledge. Additional research is sorely needed to know how to make these projects more effective. Traditional evaluation research is an integral part of the National Institute on

Drug Abuse projects, and will answer many questions about project effectiveness. In addition, we need research on outreach as *work* and as organisational activity so that we can begin to answer some of the questions raised above on these issues.

Evaluation research on outreach is not easy. In many cities, there are many different projects, and this makes it hard to assess the effects of any given one of them. Further, historical events such as the onset of new drug use patterns (cocaine injection in the late 1970s, crack in the 1980s) or the beginning of new projects during the life of an evaluation complicate analysis yet further. It is possible to try to escape these difficulties by studying the effects of randomly assigning multiple small drug-using areas to either receive the intervention or not (controls). This requires a very large number of areas to avoid statistical confounding; and contamination of control areas by travel and communication among areas remains a problem.

In spite of these difficulties, standard evaluation models do offer some insight into programme effects, and can contribute to programme design. They can let us know which approaches seem to produce no useful effects, suggest that others may be of value, and help specify which programme types are most likely to lead to risk reduction among specified types of injecting drug users or their sexual partners.

REFERENCES

Casadonte, P., Des Jarlais, D.C., Smith, T., Novatt, A. and Herndal, P. (1986) 'Psychological and behavioural impact of learning HTLV-III/LAV antibody test results', Paris: paper presented at the International Conference on AIDS.

Des Jarlais, D.C., Friedman, S.R. and Strug, D. (1986) 'AIDS and needle sharing within the intravenous drug use subculture', in D. Feldman and T. Johnson (eds) *The Social Dimensions of AIDS*, New York: Praeger.

Friedman, S.R. and Casriel, C. (1988) 'Drug users' organizations and AIDS policy', *AIDS and Public Policy* 3: 30–6.

Friedman, S.R., de Jong, W.M. and Des Jarlais, D.C. (1988) 'Problems and dynamics of organizing intravenous drug users for AIDS prevention', *Health Education Research* 3(1): 49–57.

Friedman, S.R., Des Jarlais, D.C. and Sotheran, J.L. (1986) 'AIDS health education for intravenous drug users', *Health Education Quarterly* 13: 383–94.

Friedman, S.R., Des Jarlais, D.C., Sotheran, J.L., Garber, J., Cohen, H. and Smith, D. (1987) 'AIDS and self-organization among intravenous drug users', *International Journal of the Addictions* 22(3): 201–19.

Jackson, J. and Rotkiewitz, L. (1987) 'A coupon program', Washington: paper presented at the 3rd International Conference on AIDS.

Keddie, E., Jennings, M., Jain, S., Flynn, N. and Carlson, (1988) 'Chemical inactivation of cell-associated Human Immunodeficiency Virus': paper presented at 28th Interscience Conference on Antimicrobial Agents and Chemotheraphy.

Moss, A.R. and Chaisson, R. (1988) 'AIDS and intravenous drug use in San Francisco', *AIDS and Public Policy*, 3: 37–41.

Watters, J.K. (1987) 'Preventing Human Immunodeficiency Virus contagion among intravenous drug users', Washington: paper presented at the 3rd International Conference on AIDS.

Chapter Seventeen

LOCAL COMMUNITY SERVICES

KAREN GOWLER AND GEOF RAYNER

In Britain, the development of health and social services for people with AIDS or HIV is now receiving priority attention at a time when many public services are subject to tight spending limits. However, new finance, though welcome, is only part of the picture. Despite better understanding of the clinical dimensions of AIDS, it is still too early to determine what the long-term social or public health impact of this disease will be. It is clear that HIV infection – and the growing number of people affected by it – presents a significant challenge. This is particularly true in the case of drug users and former drug users with HIV, AIDS Related Complex (ARC) or AIDS.

This chapter will examine the development of policies towards HIV and drug use in the local context. The focus will be placed upon the attitudes and practices of both mainstream services and specialist drug agencies. It is suggested that the emergence of HIV infection among drug users requires a fundamental reassessment of attitudes and practices both in specialist agencies (where they exist) and also in mainstream services, such as housing and social services. In some cases new services for drug users with HIV will be required, and while most of these will be similar to those offered to other people with HIV infection, special issues emerge which require separate consideration. One of the major lessons to be drawn from existing provision for people with AIDS is that services should be made consumer-conscious and support voluntary initiative and self-help. In order to ensure that this occurs, there may be a need to develop new means of service co-ordination, and one example is suggested. Although the institutional context discussed here relates to Britain, many issues raised will have application elsewhere. It is acknowledged that the problem of developing innovative services can be formidable. Experimentation and evaluation should therefore feature as an essential component of new provision.

WHAT IS THE DEMAND?

As yet very few drug users have been diagnosed as having AIDS in the UK, but reported HIV-antibody-positive cases continue to rise. The largest numbers are concentrated in Edinburgh, where a significant proportion of drug users are infected. In the UK, the *Report of the Working Group on Short-term Predictions of HIV Infection and AIDS in England and Wales* (*Cox Report*) was issued at the end of 1988, predicting a mounting overall caseload. Using Cox's figures, one Regional Health Authority, North West Thames, gauged that they needed to plan for a four-fold rise in community care services for people with AIDS by 1992. Services therefore have only a small breathing space in which to plan new services for people already infected. With regard to drug users with HIV, some lessons have already been learnt in provision of services to people with AIDS from other groups, including the need for a planned, co-ordinated response. However, provision of services for drug users may present many more difficulties. Some of these relate to drug misuse, but an additional problem concerns the way drug users are viewed by society.

THE OFFICIAL RESPONSE TO HIV/AIDS

Action on drugs and HIV has to be seen in context, both in terms of how national policy has developed and also how people with drugs problems or with AIDS are viewed in local communities. Nationally, the British Department of Health, along with the Health Education Authority, have invested considerable resources in educating the general public about HIV. Although these educational initiatives suffered some political interference, they did not succumb to politically-defined moral imperatives (specifically, exhortations to chastity, monogamy and heterosexuality) which would have blunted the public health message. However, questions can still be raised over the effectiveness of the campaign. For example, while the gay community has reduced risk-taking behaviour (shown through the spectacular reduction in sexually transmitted infections among this group), health education initiatives directed at the heterosexual population (including drug users) have been of limited success. In response, beginning in November 1988, a new campaign was developed. Aimed at drug users, it focused on the risks of injecting drugs and sharing needles and syringes.

In terms of local provision, the situation is perhaps less clear-cut because services vary enormously from one place to another. Until recently, considerable attention – and finance – has been focused upon the clinical dimensions of treatment of people with AIDS, ARC or HIV, usually within the hospital setting. However, the need to develop a community-based model of service has been recognised, and former Secretary of State for Social Services Norman Fowler visited agencies in San Francisco and New York City in 1986. However, the services that Fowler saw were mainly for gay men, not for drug users. People affected by HIV in San Francisco are a relatively homogeneous – mostly gay – and a politically influential and generally affluent group. They are located in an unusually accepting social setting. Where there is experience in developing new services for people with HIV who are drug users, the picture is rather depressing. The American city with the largest proportion of people with HIV is New York. Here, a growing proportion are drug users; most are black and poor. Self-organisation among drug users with AIDS is practically non-existent. Many are isolated from families or friendship networks. Most face exclusion from mainstream services; indeed, for many their main contact with state authorities is with law enforcement agencies. Unlike San Francisco, a growing proportion of those affected are women, who may be drug users or the sexual partners of drug users with HIV. AIDS has been typified as a major crisis for the gay community, yet its impact on heterosexual drug users poses different – and, in some ways, greater – challenges. While the model of voluntary, self-help activity in San Francisco is important, it requires specification in the British context.

MODELS OF CARE FOR DRUG USERS WITH HIV

The issue of defining a model of care for drug users with HIV has so far received little attention, which may be due to the tendency to view the needs of drug users solely in terms of their addiction to drugs. However, drug users with HIV share some common attributes with some of the established need groups with whom the concept of community care has usually been established. Although other groups – such as the disabled – would probably resent the comparison, they too share stigmatisation. How somebody came to be infected with HIV has no bearing on the community services they require at the onset of illness. Good housing, financial support, help in the home, and social and emotional support are the basic needs of anybody with AIDS or other severe health problems. Therefore, the services developed for people with AIDS should cater for all those affected, regardless of how they came in contact with the virus. Drug users may have more acute needs for community services, as they may not have a secure place to live or may not have any network of informal support. They may also require specialist help in relation to their drug use. Community services must be planned in partnership with acute hospital services, specialist drug agencies, the voluntary sector and self-help organisations. If one link in this complex chain of support is lacking, the other elements will increasingly be unable to cope. In order to ensure that people with HIV or AIDS come forward to obtain services, their confidentiality needs to be assured.

Specialist drug services

Some questions have to be aimed at the specialist drug agencies. For example, how far do drug prevention and treatment efforts need to change? Should drug agencies provide a different type of service for clients with HIV? Specialist drug services have so far had limited acquaintance with HIV/AIDS, and either there is confusion over the direction of services or perhaps worse, a head-in-the-sand attitude towards AIDS. One key problem concerns whom drug services cater for. Generally speaking, this is a minority of drug users. The enduring reality is that many people either at risk of HIV, or some proportion of those already infected (and who may not know that they are infected), may not be in contact with any service. Drug users and ex-drug users are often discriminated against or ignored, sometimes because of fear and ignorance, and sometimes because their problems are seen as self-inflicted. Many are not experienced in the use of services, and while some drug users may have regular contact with the medical profession, this may be limited to drug dependence units. Drug agencies are not experienced in providing assistance to users with HIV. Furthermore, someone may be viewed as a drug user first, and a person with HIV second.

This dilemma concerning the relative importance of drug use *vis-à-vis* HIV infection also produces conundrums for drug treatment services based upon the concept of a therapeutic community (see Chapter 23). For example, a service which emphasises total abstinence from drugs by implication tends to emphasise the drug problem (which, for most, is not a life-long condition) rather than HIV (which is). Drug users may become ill during treatment and may be traumatised by what many consider to be a life-threatening disease.

General services

Specialisation by drug agencies around the 'problems' of the drug user may have led many people working in generic services to consider themselves unqualified to deal with the problems faced by drug users and ex-users, and even less qualified in cases where HIV infection is involved. However, many local authorities are providing community services such as home helps, advice on financial assistance and are attempting to solve housing difficulties for people with AIDS (Bebbington and Warren 1988). Some have initiated ambitious staff training programmes to dispel fears and discrimination around AIDS. Due to the mystery, anxiety and ignorance surrounding drugs, drug users with AIDS may be seen as a more difficult group to help. The perceptions of drug users do powerfully shape the way services are offered. Mutual suspicion exists on both sides. Some metropolitan social services departments which may have adopted an enlightened stance towards gay men with AIDS may still retain stereotypes about drug users; parents who use drugs often have fears that their children will be taken into care if they seek help – fears that have been aggravated by recent highly publicised court decisions. There is a role for 'awareness raising' in mainstream services. Specialist drug agencies and self-help groups could be involved in providing the support for clients and the necessary training and education for staff working in community services.

Homelessness and housing

It must be emphasised that even if attitudes are changed, the practical issues of developing services are legion. Many drug users who become ill as a result of HIV infection will be homeless or living in poor housing. In New York City, where the problems of homelessness are acute, the AIDS Resource Center, in collaboration with the City Administration, has developed scattered site housing and a 45-bed residential facility for people with AIDS – most of whom are former drug users. In Britain, some local authority housing departments are viewing symptomatic HIV as a criterion for rehousing. However, pressure on local authority housing departments, especially in London, has led to many homeless families living in bed and breakfast accommodation for months and even years before being offered permanent housing. Single people come well down the list of priorities: they may be offered bed and breakfast or hostel accommodation or, somewhat better, a hard-to-let flat. The new housing legislation is likely to make matters worse. This does not mean that this option should not be explored, but it is realistic to assume that even those authorities which claim to offer enlightened policies are hardly in a position to deliver on their promises.

Some of the best practice in housing provision, particularly for groups with special needs, has been through the voluntary housing sector. However, most housing associations may feel uncertain about developing a special project for this controversial client group, and in any case projects for AIDS are competing against other priorities. Furthermore, the financial arrangements governing special projects, already beset by difficulties, are subject to continued uncertainty. The Department of Health considers housing to be an important part of the continuum of care, but the guidelines for housing finance are set by the Department of the Environment, whose sympathies towards this client group are yet to be revealed. Clearly, extra finance needs to be made available through the Housing Corporation, and consideration given to the extra expense of developing housing provision for people who may become severely ill and housebound.

While finance is a major issue, there is still the judgement to be made about the kind of housing provision that should be developed (Resource Information Service 1987). In 1984, when

AIDS first gained public attention in Britain, the idea of AIDS 'hospices' became the vogue. However, although special facilities have developed for the severely ill – for example, the Mildmay Hospital and the London Lighthouse (which is a multi-purpose organisation) – experience from the USA as well as from Britain suggests that hospices may have only limited applicability, since people with AIDS experience a typically episodic pattern of illness, from being at the verge of death at one moment to relative well-being at another. The best assumption to make is that most people will want a home of their own (and some will wish to die at home), and that services should be delivered to them as appropriate. Practically, then, housing schemes should be developed in close association with social services departments and health services community units. In London, there are several schemes being developed. Strutton Housing Association is a specialist housing association developing scattered site accommodation. The criterion for access to a Strutton house is homelessness. Another scheme being developed in London is associated with the Landmark (a charity for people with HIV and AIDS), whose *raison d'être* is the co-ordination of statutory and voluntary services. The Landmark model is based upon the clustering of separate flats, testing the notion that some of the people who are touched by this illness can share mutual support. Anything larger than, say, six places means an institutional form of provision, or goes ahead on the assumption that the project would have special characteristics which would overcome this problem (for example, the project may offer a high level of nursing support or comprise a residential therapeutic community).

Drug users with families have long been wary of contact with either the health service or social services, particularly given the high degree of sensitivity afforded to child abuse. This problem needs to be overcome. For parents who are HIV positive this will cause them great concern about their relationships with their children; they will wonder whether to tell their children about the nature of their illness, and how they will cope when they are unwell. It is therefore particularly important that this burden is shared with sympathetic outsiders, whether they are professional staff, befrienders or others. Having a social worker is a gateway to other forms of service and advice. Social services departments are now issuing guidelines on the response to families or to children with HIV infection, as well as publicising policies on confidentiality. The Advisory Council on the Misuse of Drugs (1988) has recommended that social services departments work to ensure that 'drug misuse alone does not constitute grounds for taking a child into care and neither does HIV infection. The usual criteria applied to child care should be used and the parents' behaviour in relation to the child should be the priority consideration.' Social services policies in London and Edinburgh are based on guidelines for anti-discrimination; however, it would be false to make confident assertions about services elsewhere. Importantly, local authority associations are attempting to standardise models of good practice.

NEW PRINCIPLES FOR SERVICES

Hopefully, the pressure exerted on statutory agencies to develop new services in the light of demand projections will create a new environment. Adjusting to HIV among drug users calls for a radical overhaul of attitudes and practices, but on what principle does this task begin?

The first principle is controversial. HIV antibody status is more important than drug use status. In consequence, services should be matched to the HIV problem first, with drug use placed second. Indeed, the issue of drug use itself may be somewhere down the list of problems faced by the client: lack of housing, income, or social supports may be more pressing.

A second principle concerns the planning of provision. Experience of the working of drug advisory committees, the link between statutory and voluntary services (health, police, local authorities, etc.), suggests they have not adjusted to HIV, whereas some of the new mechanisms of co-ordination – the variously titled HIV working parties – explicitly have. This does not mean that drug advisory committees should be abandoned, but they must accept a much wider brief or alternative mechanisms will need to be developed.

Having said that HIV should become the primary focus for services, this does not mean a downgrading of the importance of specialist drug agencies. However, they have much to learn about the workings of other services – services with which they perhaps have had little contact in the past. If the focus is to be on the client's needs and not just on the 'drug problem', then it follows that a client's difficulties may be linked to housing, health care, isolation from social supports, and other factors. If drug users are excluded from mainstream services, specialist drug agencies may wish to examine the sort of support they feel they should offer. In Britain, most drug agencies are small, and while they may consider providing housing, welfare rights or social services advice, they are not likely to perform this task effectively. A better approach would seem to be for each agency to be fully aware of what local services are available and to develop contact with them.

Drug users may not have a network of friends and family to turn to for support and may need help from a wide range of services from different authorities. The issue of friendship networks for drug users is a perplexing one. People who are long-term drug users may have developed friendships based on drug dealing and using. One of the tasks of developing personally supportive arrangements for individuals is that of helping drug users to recognise the limitations of these networks and how to develop alternatives. The development of the therapeutic community model of drug rehabilitation has in part this objective. In terms of seeking support from existing services, including drugs services, the problem is that, to repeat an earlier point, even the most enlightened provider may view the HIV-positive user as a drug user first, and a person with other needs second. To use one typical example, a general practitioner may narrowly visualise the needs of a drug user as drugs-related and ignore other dimensions of health and illness.

Part of the interest in services in San Francisco concerned the use of volunteers. In Britain, too, the 'buddy' or befriending system has played an important role in providing much-needed support to people isolated and traumatised by a diagnosis of HIV or AIDS (see Chapter 22). But while volunteers can complement hospital and community services, they cannot replace them; volunteering should best be seen as one component of a philosophy of self-help whereby the affected groups look to resources within themselves to develop a collective response to illness. However, it is important both to understand its purposes as well as limitations. Self-help in the context of HIV and AIDS means the development of mutual support systems; it does not mean individuals or groups turn their back on what statutory services have to offer (see

Chapter 22). In Britain, groups like Body Positive and Frontliners (mainly composed of gay men) have developed autonomously to provide mutual support, and newer groups are being formed – Positively Women and Mainliners (for drug users) are two examples.

Although drug users may not be predisposed to act in common interest this is certainly not true of *former* drug users. Former drug users compose some of the most knowledgeable and empathic drug workers, and because they provide a role model to people attempting to come off drugs, they are likely to be the most effective. Groups like Mainliners will therefore have an extremely important role to play in supporting drug users with HIV, in regards to coming to terms with drugs as well as HIV. These groups should be the natural allies of professional staff, but will only become so if the latter display professional flexibility in their methods and philosophy.

One outstanding issue which will be resolved only in the light of experience will be whether some of the newer provisions for people with HIV will be able to encompass the diversity of expressed needs. Or, put slightly differently, will different groups of people be sympathetic to each other? In South London, this question has been raised in what some regard as a model service. The Landmark integrates some of the best aspects of statutory and voluntary services. It aims to provide support and advice to all people with HIV infection and to act as a referral, information and co-ordination point for social and community health services across several boroughs and health authorities. A key objective of the centre is to help make statutory services work for people with HIV in order for them to continue as normal a life as possible. The centre opened in 1989 and forms a base for some of those services and also organises volunteers, education, outreach work and will manage supported housing. It will also train workers in statutory agencies and help ease the communications difficulties which frequently occur as well as develop a 'knowledge base' or who does what – for example, on which days environmental health staff collect infectious waste, and how to find short-cuts through red tape. As regards drug users, the centre has formal links via an HIV/drugs worker, with a drug street agency and a syringe-exchange scheme. However, the new centre acknowledges this may not be enough. Charting a course for a service for everyone requires utmost sensitivity, and it remains to be seen whether such a broad-based service, helping a wide range of people, will succeed in its aims.

Until recently in Britain, it was acknowledged that there existed a breathing-space in which to develop a response to HIV and AIDS. That space has now closed. Much effort is going into developing new services and ensuring that people with HIV or AIDS are provided with existing services in ways which avoid discrimination. However, most existing practice is based upon metropolitan settings, where the scale of the issue means that specialist services can develop. In smaller communities, the task will be that much more difficult. It is therefore extremely important that all agencies involved in developing new services, or revising what they do at present, honestly appraise their difficulties.

REFERENCES

Advisory Council on the Misuse of Drugs (1988) *AIDS and Drug Misuse Report: Part II*, London: Department of Health.

Bebbington, A. and Warren, P. (1988) AIDS: *The Local Authority Response*, University of Kent: Canterbury Personal Social Services Research Unit.

Resource Information Service (1987) *AIDS: The Issues for Housing*, London.

Working Group on Short-term Predictions of HIV Infection and AIDS in England and Wales (1988) *Report*, London: HMSO.

Chapter Eighteen

HIV INFECTION AND AIDS IN THE PRISON ENVIRONMENT: A TEST CASE FOR THE RESPECT OF HUMAN RIGHTS

TIMOTHY HARDING

In considering the responses to the drug taker in the prison environment, the humane and generous values implied in the title of this book encounter hard realities. These reveal society's ambivalence towards the problems of drug users and remind us that there is a real risk that the efforts to combat the AIDS epidemic by applying well-established public health principles and respecting fundamental ethical values concerning personal autonomy, relief of suffering and promotion of health, can be undermined and replaced by other sinister reactions based on fear and rejection. Experience has shown that the drug taker is especially at risk of non-respect of basic human rights – and nowhere more than in prisons. This chapter is imbued with a sense of doubt and warning. The overall impression of the management of HIV and AIDS in prisons is pessimistic. Opportunities are being missed; counselling for seropositive prisoners is insufficient; care for prisoners with AIDS is inadequate; prison administrations and judicial authorities are unprepared for the complex decisions which must be taken concerning both individuals and institutions.

Public health policy concerning HIV infection is based on information to the public designed to promote responsible behaviour. Repressive measures of control – in particular, obligatory screening, segregation and isolation – are thought to be unnecessary and counterproductive. Respect for human rights and ethical principles has therefore become a major element in the global effort to control the HIV epidemic.

Prisons are a place where the defence of human rights assumes special importance. Applying public health policy on HIV infection and AIDS in the prison environment can therefore be regarded as a test case in the respect for human rights of the individual, whether that individual is infected or not.

Health authorities were initially slow to react to the AIDS problem in prisons. In many countries, preventive health and medical care in prisons are administered separately from community health services. Standards of medical care in prisons are frequently criticised. Ethical issues of professional independence, confidentiality and consent to treatment remain unresolved. Hygiene standards legally required in the community are not uniformly applied in prisons.

In the summer of 1985, serious disturbances took place in many European prisons. Staff and inmates had learnt that AIDS had not spared prisons. The authorities seemed unprepared. Initial reactions mirrored uncertainty and concern in the whole community, but were amplified by the closed, authoritarian environment of prisons where rumours and suspicion thrive.

This chapter is based on impressions gained, as well as data collected, during a study on AIDS in the member states of the Council of Europe. The study was carried out in 1987 and updated in 1988. The results have been presented in a report published by the Council of Europe (1987) and summarised in an article (Harding 1987). Drawing attention to the problem of HIV and AIDS in prison has had complex and unpredictable side-effects. The linking of AIDS and prisons in titles of articles or of consultations has tended to create the false impression that prison is a major risk factor in the AIDS epidemic and that exceptional measures are justified. Controversy has become focused on single issues, especially the availability of condoms in prisons (McMillan 1988). Prisons are portrayed as a world apart whereas there is in fact a constant flow between prisons and the general population.

The growing number of drug users in Europe's prisons over the past 20 years has meant that prisons are now the single largest response to the drug problem in most European countries. More resources are deployed in processing drug users through the criminal justice system and housing them in prisons than on any other form of management, whether medical or social. This option had already created a sense of failure and missed opportunities in helping drug users, even before AIDS. One should not therefore be surprised at the way in which prison systems have reacted to the epidemic. Muddling through, inconsistency and lack of forward planning would be relatively mild expressions of the inadequacies.

The clear and useful recommendations of the World Health Organization consultation on the control of AIDS in prisons (1987) reflect a straightforward principle: health care within prisons should be equivalent to health care in the community. This would be translated into preventive action based on information, the respect of the individual, counselling and human care. In addition, one would hope to be able to use the prison as an opportunity for active health education, counselling and helping inmates prepare for release.

While these opportunities exist, the clear impression from contacts with prison medical services in many countries is that segregation and stigmatisation of seropositive prisoners is common, information provided to staff and inmates is incomplete and sometimes counterproductive and little or no counselling is available.

HIV SEROPOSITIVITY IN EUROPE'S PRISONS

Risk factors

Several factors increase the probability of prisoners being seropositive on entry, in comparison to the general population. The first is the extent of injecting drug use among prisoners. Available figures from France, Holland, Switzerland, Italy and Spain indicate that, during the three months prior to entry, 20–30 per cent of prisoners have regularly (at least once a week) injected drugs. This is without doubt the single most important risk factor and provides a sufficient explanation for the epidemiological observations. Second, there is the demographic structure of the prison population. Prisoners are predominantly young men. The mean age in European prisons varies from 27 to 33 years by country. Between 85 and 95 per cent per cent of inmates are men. Over 80 per cent of prisoners are in the age range 18 to 40 years. Prison populations therefore correspond closely to the demographic distribution of the risk groups for HIV infection in the general population of European countries. Third, there is sexual promiscuity. There is no evidence that prisoners prior to entry have a sexual life-style which is more promiscuous than the general population. In fact, opiate abuse probably diminishes sexual drive. However, acute gonorrhoea and serological evidence of syphilis are commoner in prisoners on entry than in the general population. A significant proportion of women prisoners display two behavioural risk factors: intravenous drug abuse (e.g. 60 per cent of female prisoners in Swiss prisons) and regular or intermittent prostitution. Finally, in relation to homosexuality, there is no clear data on the frequency of a homosexual or bisexual orientation among prisoners, prior to entry. Homosexual contacts occur in prison, and well-documented cases of sexually transmitted diseases other than HIV have been reported among prisoners, such that transmission must have occurred in prison.

Surveys of HIV seropositivity

There is now considerable evidence about HIV seropositivity in European prisons. Small-scale studies on samples of prisoners reveal that, among 500 consecutive entries in a French prison serving a mainly urban area, HIV seropositivity was almost exclusively associated with injecting drug abuse and found in 12.6 per cent of entries. In Switzerland, the total population of inmates in adult prison establishments in the canton of Berne (n=387) showed an HIV seroprevalence of 11 per cent. In Holland, a survey in the central Amsterdam prison, with a high proportion of injecting drug users, indicated an overall seropositivity rate of 11 per cent. In Italy, of over 30,000 prisoners screened on entry in 1986, 16 per cent were seropositive. Finally, in Spain, screening programmes have demonstrated that over 25 per cent of male prisoners were seropositive.

It seems reasonable to infer that in European countries more than 10 per cent of prisoners are seropositive – overall, 30,000 seropositive prisoners. However, the frequency is variable, with some countries having rates in the region of 1–2 per cent (Belgium and Luxembourg) and others even lower (Portugal, <0.1 per cent); Cyprus, 0 per cent). In other countries (Ireland, UK, Sweden and Austria) the data are difficult to interpret.

The factors which appear to determine the rate of seropositivity among prisoners in a given country are the proportion of prisoners who were injecting drug abusers prior to imprisonment, and the rate of seropositivity among injecting drug abusers in the community.

In fact, the prevalence of HIV seropositivity among prisoners has little epidemiological importance. The AIDS epidemic has simply revealed the vulnerability of the prison population in general and the adverse consequences of a public policy which has led to the criminalisation and penalisation of the problem of drug dependence. There are very many drug-dependent persons in Europe's prisons. Many of these persons are HIV seropositive and will develop AIDS. The prison environment must respond to this challenge. The underlying question is whether the response will correspond to generally accepted scientific, ethical and humanitarian standards.

SPECIAL SIGNIFICANCE OF HIV IN PRISON

Epidemiological bridging

Prisons may well occupy a key position for the control of HIV in the community. They provide a 'bridging situation', where considerable numbers of injecting drug users (a high proportion of whom are HIV carriers) can be expected to have occasional homosexual contacts. The frequency and type of homosexual contacts in prison are not known, but anecdotal accounts by prisoners suggest that anal intercourse and mouth/genital sex are rather frequent, even between prisoners who have heterosexual orientation outside prison. A report from American prisons indicates that 19 per cent of prisoners serving sentences of six months or over report at least one homosexual contact while in prison. Thus, induced homosexual behaviour in prison provides a 'bridge' between a known high-risk group (injecting drug abusers) and individuals who may later become a source of infection through heterosexual contacts. It is vital to limit this bridging phenomenon which may contribute to the spread of HIV.

Risk of transmission via needles and syringes

The risk of HIV transmission as a result of injecting drug use among prisoners is difficult to assess. There is no doubt that the frequency of injectable drug use among opiate-dependent persons is lower in prison than in the community. However, when heroin is smuggled into the prison, clean needles and syringes are not available. Inevitably, drug-dependent prisoners will share a needle and syringe, without adequate sterilisation. The overall risk is therefore probably at least as high in prisons as in the community. Three types of response to this risk have been suggested:

i The reinforcement of security measures to limit the extent of drug smuggling. Such measures inevitably create increased tension and mistrust, through regular body searches, restrictions on parcels, books and other materials sent from outside and limiting strictly any direct contact with visitors.

ii The provision of needles and syringes to prisons on the same basis as in the community. This raises extremely difficult problems of discipline and of coherence in the attitudes of the prison authorities. Virtually all prison authorities have indicated that such a solution is 'unthinkable'.

iii The reduction of the risk of heroin abuse by methadone maintenance treatment programmes in prison. This approach is currently being assessed in New York's prison system. It raises extremely difficult issues, both practical and ethical, concerning the selection of patient and follow-up treatment after release.

At the very least, needle and syringe availability should be discussed for open prisons where inmates work in the community, for periods of trial release and at the time of final release.

Pressure for obligatory control measures

The fact that it is possible to impose much stricter controls in the prisons has led to suggestions that strict controls should be imposed to limit the spread of HIV. Such a policy would imply compulsory testing of all prisoners for HIV antibodies. The 'paternalistic' approach can be defended by arguing that prison authorities have a direct responsibility to protect prisoners from the consequences of promiscuity; the possibility of homosexual rape in prisons is real. Nevertheless, there is a clear impression that those who advocate routine, compulsory screening of prisoners are seeking a scapegoat group for political reasons. If a significant risk of homosexual rape exists in prisons, this is an argument for improving human conditions for prisoners and staff/prisoner ratios, decreasing overcrowding and providing activities rather than for imposing compulsory screening with no safeguards on confidentiality.

Psychological reactions

Persons who are told that they are HIV seropositive react characteristically by an initial period of denial and disbelief. Some ask for the test to be repeated. There follows a period of emotional lability, accompanied by an urgent need to communicate and discuss. Acute depression and suicide attempts may occur, since friends and family are not available. Characteristic feelings and reactions expressed by prisoners are:

Defence mechanisms:	'Everyone must die some day.' 'My body is strong, I will beat the virus.' 'A treatment will be found soon.' 'The epidemic is exaggerated.'
Fatalism:	'My life was already rotten.' 'AIDS is the last of my problems.' 'If I have to die . . . why not?'
Guilt:	Particularly concerning former sexual partners and unborn children.
Anger:	'If I am seropositive, I don't care whom I infect.'

Depressed feelings about decreased life-expectancy are heightened in prisoners by the sense of injustice and impotence: 'If I have only a few years to live, why should I spend them inside?' Fears are also expressed about developing AIDS while in prison. Other prisoners accept the decreased life-expectancy with equanimity but are devastated by the thought that they cannot have children. Perhaps the most painful experience for HIV-seropositive prisoners is the fear expressed by staff, fellow-prisoners and their family and the experience of being rejected by friends, neighbours and other social contacts.

FEAR VERSUS TRUST: PROBLEMS OF HEALTH EDUCATION IN A CLOSED ENVIRONMENT

Health education must be based on trust; the prison environment undermines trust. Attempts to develop HIV health education are handicapped by several features of the prison environment and experience.

First, prisons are grim places: they are overcrowded, sordidly unhygienic and house inmates with high rates of chronic social problems, personality disorders and psychiatric illness. Fears and suspicion abound; information circulates through rumours and confidences. Common occurrences in European prisons are: self-mutilation, mainly wrist slashing; fist fights and other forms of physical violence leading to open wounds and bleeding; slops (bucketfuls of urine and faeces kept overnight in cells) overturned, spilt or thrown at guards or other prisoners; casual homosexual contacts (mutual masturbation, orogenital sex, sodomy) practised by men with a heterosexual orientation outside prison. Such prisoners lack the vocabulary and knowledge needed to assimilate information about 'safer sex' practices. Discussing this kind of homosexuality is extremely difficult in view of the associated shame and guilt; tattooing is often practised by prisoners with homemade materials. It is not easy under such conditions to carry out effective health education about AIDS, based on open, frank communication. It is even less easy if prisoners perceive the prison medical staff as belonging to the system, an integral part of the prison hierarchy.

Second, cognitive problems among prisoners make communication of essential information about AIDS difficult. Such problems include: lack of reading skills; language difficulties; intellectual limitations and attention deficits created by stressful conditions. Depression and suicide are common among prisoners, especially during the remand phase (see studies by Blackett 1987; Clavel *et al.* 1987). Prisoners are preoccupied and stressed. Can AIDS education be counterproductive in such circumstances? In particular, might HIV testing do harm? Carefully monitored pilot studies are required to identify the balance of benefit and cost of such interventions. Is prison really a good place for young drug addicts to learn of their HIV seropositivity? Without the support of family and friends, already subject to stress, the drug addict is faced with an intolerable additional burden. Suicide attempts in prison immediately after the communication of test results are not uncommon. Other prisoners use denial as a mechanism of defence, which negates the effect of health education.

Third, if seropositive prisoners suffer from discrimination, overtly or covertly, in contacts with other prisoners, access to workshops or leisure activities, this will undermine health education designed to demonstrate the specificity of transmission routes.

Most people entering prison stay for a period of not more than six months. Health education should be aimed not only at reducing risk during the prison stay, but should also prepare the individual for release – particularly in the case of the young drug users. If there is too great a discordance between conditions in prisons and the community (e.g. availability of condoms, syringes and needles) the information becomes incoherent.

PRISONERS WHO DEVELOP AIDS

At the end of 1986, 32 cases of AIDS had been diagnosed according to a study of the prisons of 17 European countries. All had occurred in two countries: Italy (10 cases) and Spain (22 cases). At the end of 1987, a partial survey through contact with prison medical services in 11 countries revealed that over 100 new cases had been diagnosed in the intervening 12 months. Countries reporting cases at the end of 1987 included: Austria, Belgium, Federal Republic of Germany, France, Holland, Italy, Spain, Sweden and Switzerland. In addition, there are now at least 300 prisoners with AIDS Related Complex (ARC) in the same countries.

A five- to ten-fold increase in the incidence of AIDS cases among prisoners is predicted over the next three years.

Measures already taken include:

- specially adapted prison regimes (improved diet, light work, better physical conditions) for prisoners with ARC syndrome and early stages of AIDS;
- treatment in prison hospitals or prison wards in general hospitals;
- transfer to general hospitals with surveillance;
- suspension of sentence in the final stages of illness, with repatriation in the case of foreigners.

Problems encountered in the management of prisoners with AIDS include:

— increased risk of opportunistic infections for ARC and AIDS patients in the prison environment;
— difficulty in managing behavioural symptoms (confusion, withdrawal, bizarre behaviour) in AIDS patients with Central Nervous System involvement;
— problems in giving accurate prognosis to judicial authorities;
— difficulty of securing release for prisoners on remand;
— access for family members during acute and terminal phase of the illness;
— lack of health insurance for prisoners released on compassionate grounds.

Once again, we can define a common denominator to these problems: an underlying conflict of values between the penal system (based on the principles of 'just deserts', retribution and dissuasion) and medical care (based on promoting health and limiting suffering). Young drug-dependent prisoners are already stigmatised and marginalised. What chances do they have of receiving humane care throughout the period of the illness, including the terminal phase?

CONCLUSION

The high prevalence of seropositivity and the rising incidence of AIDS among prisoners is a direct reflection of the number of injecting drug abusers in prison populations. Prisons should not be regarded *per se* as a risk factor for HIV infection or AIDS. Transmission between drug users by needle sharing exists in prison as elsewhere, with the added factor of non-availability of syringes. A potential risk of epidemiological bridging by induced homosexual behaviour exists in prison, but transmission of HIV in such circumstances has only recently been demonstrated.

Prison conditions make health education difficult. Psychological reactions are especially serious and difficult to manage among seropositive prisoners. It is also clear that in many countries, medical confidentiality is not guaranteed, and prison administrators receive HIV antibody test results. Measures taken in these countries (routine isolation, restricted access to prison workshops) have no scientific basis. At the same time as these unjustifiable, unnecessary and counterproductive measures are enforced, the preventive measures recommended for the general populations – in particular, the use of condoms in casual sexual contacts – are denied to prisoners.

We can conclude that ethical and scientific standards in the control of HIV and care of AIDS in prison do not correspond to those accepted for the community in general. Improvements are unlikely unless the structure of health care delivery to prisoners is radically changed by greater independence and more resources.

REFERENCES

Blackett, S.A. (1987) 'Suicide in Scottish prisons', *British Journal of Psychiatry*, 151: 218–21.

Clavel, F., Benhamou, S. and Flamant, R. (1987) 'Decreased mortality among male prisoners', *Lancet* ii: 1012–14.

Council of Europe (1987) *Health Problems Facing Prison Administrations with Special Reference to Transmissible Diseases*, Strasbourg: Council of Europe.

Harding, T.W. (1987) 'AIDS in prison', *Lancet* ii: 1260–3.

McMillan, A. (1988) 'HIV in prisons: action, research and condoms needed', *British Medical Journal* 297: 873–4.

World Health Organization (1987) *Prevention and Control of AIDS in Prison: Recommendations of a Consultation*, Geneva: World Health Organization.

Part Five

RESPONDING: CHANGING PRACTICE

Chapter Nineteen

INTERMEDIATE GOALS AND THE PROCESS OF CHANGE

JOHN STRANG

If drug workers were bus conductors, the 'problem' would be public transport. For the planners, there would be a need to ensure that buses ran along various different routes according to timetables which took note of popular times and popular journeys. Extra buses would be required during the rush hour and on well-established link routes; and sometimes the extra capacity of double-decker buses would be important. If the public transport is being run as a public service and not just on a 'for profit' basis, then there would also be a need for occasional rural routes and late-night buses.

And how does the service seem from the point of view of the would-be travellers? They need to be able to identify the bus as their required transport when it comes along. They cannot reasonably expect the bus to come along immediately or to pick them up from their own front door, but they might just be lucky (in which case they are far more likely to use public transport regularly). If the bus stop is too far or the wait too long, then they will seek alternative transport – either their own cars from out of the garage, a car-share or a more expensive but readily available taxi.

There are some further important considerations to the running of the service. If the service is to be valuable, then it should be sufficiently clean and attractive that passengers will choose to continue using it until they reach their journey's end. If there are excessive delays or disruptions, passengers may decide to get off before they reach their destination. Perhaps more annoying than a bus that does not arrive on time is one that drives past full; consequently, it is important that people get off the bus once they reach their destination so as to make way for new passengers. The planners can reasonably expect most passengers to fit in, to a certain extent, with the collective nature of the service; but if their public service is insufficiently available or too highly priced, then the would-be traveller may opt for the ubiquitous black taxi – higher priced but always cruising around and hence readily available.

However, we are not bus conductors, and there are important differences which must be recognised in the operation of a public treatment service for drug users. We have views on which journeys we should encourage the drug user to contemplate and enact (e.g. to non-injectible drug use and/or to abstinence) and which journeys we should actively discourage (e.g. the journey from smoking to injecting). There will be those who seek a particular treatment (e.g. out-patient prescribing) for whom we believe that the treatment would not be beneficial in the long term (e.g. by virtue of previous failed journeys) and for whom we would wish to offer a different, more challenging treatment approach; thus, our energies may be directed into active promotion of a less popular journey with drug users for whom that particular journey may be especially beneficial.

MOTIVATION TO CHANGE

The argument has been put forward that there need to be different services according to the different levels of motivation of the drug taker. The ensuing discussions are often handicapped by reliance on a simplistic concept of motivation in which motivation is either present or absent. By mistakenly assuming that the drug taker can be categorically assigned to 'motivated', or 'unmotivated' it might then seem appropriate to consider separately the service needs of the 'motivated' and the 'unmotivated'. However, once the non-categorical nature of motivation is recognised, then it becomes clear that drug services need to consider ways of engaging drug takers at different points on the continuum of motivation to change, rather than acting like Procrustes and forcing the drug taker to fit the pre-formed mould of the service. In reality, motivation is not a simple on/off phenomenon but exists in varying degrees of strength for each of many possible goals. The degree of motivation will obviously depend on the goal in question and will vary from one individual to the next; it will also vary within one individual over time. Strength of motivation to change may be enhanced or diminished by pressure (or the lack of it) from family or friends, the courts, and – crucially – by drug treatment services themselves. These drug treatment services must come to recognise that they are part of the phenomenon which they seek to observe; and thus they must look for ways to maximise the beneficial effect of their contact with the drug taker, rather than just sitting back and dispassionately (or passionately) observing the phenomena. These considerations become all the more urgent when the HIV issue is taken into account. Drug services must now adopt a more pro-active role and 'make contact with a much larger proportion of drug misusers and work with them to change their behaviour', as recommended by the Advisory Council on the Misuse of Drugs in their report on *AIDS and Drug Misuse* (1988). As yet, they are rarely able to respond to the call from the US Presidential Commission on the Human Immunodeficiency Virus Epidemic (1988) that there should be 'treatment on demand'.

THE PROCESS OF CHANGE

A dilemma exists with the prescribing of drugs such as opiates. In the drug field, prescribing might best be considered as an agent that enables some other change to take place. Change must be recognised as a process of adaptation rather than as a simple one-off event: it follows that there will be factors which increase or decrease the likelihood of movement through the process, and factors which influence the speed of this movement. The benefit or otherwise of a particular intervention is probably not intrinsic, but is only evident when considered for an individual drug taker according to the extent to which it promotes or impedes movement through the process of change.

Prochaska and Di Clemente (1986) have described a theoretical model for understanding the process of change (see Figure 19.1). The pre-contemplative drug taker may be prompted by positive or negative reinforcing factors to consider the benefits and costs of the present behaviour compared to some altered circumstances. These influences may be the identification of benefit associated with a change or may alternatively be a realisation of the adverse

Figure 19.1 The process of change

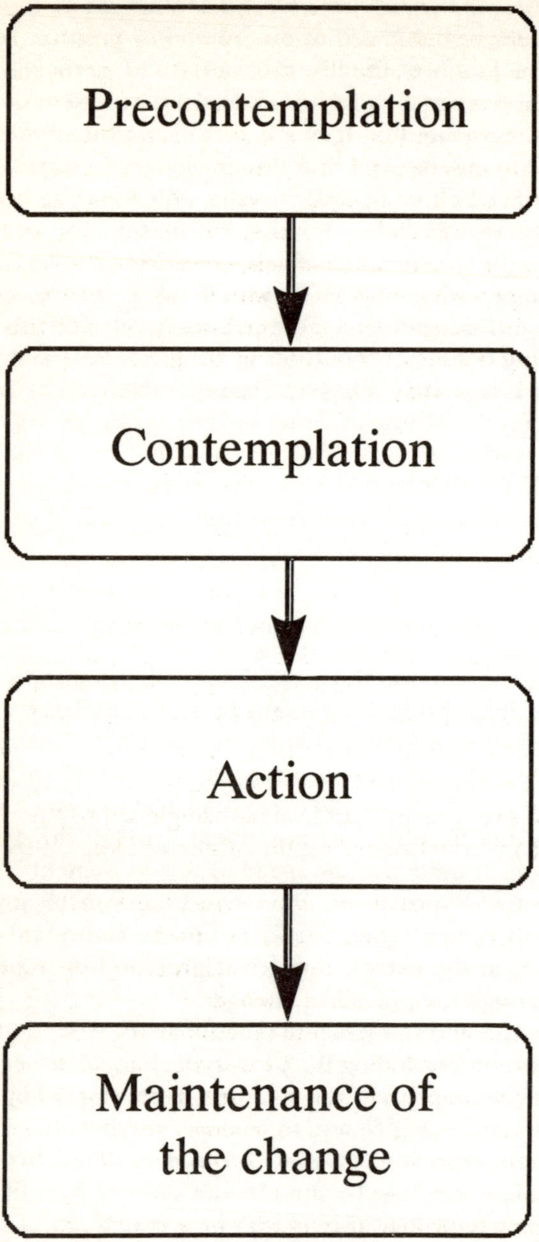

consequences of continuation of the present behaviour. In the stage of contemplation, the drug user is actively conducting a cost–benefit analysis, and some drug workers will now help the drug taker to undertake this analysis with separate consideration of the short-term and long-term benefits and consequences. The extent of movement on to the stage of action (i.e. implementing the change) may be markedly influenced by the availability of help to bring about the changes – availability locally and at time of need. Having effected a change, the drug taker will again be conducting a cost–benefit analysis, comparing the costs and benefits of the present new situation with those of a return to drug use.

What influence does prescribing have on this process? Prescribing does not directly bring about the beneficial change – rather, it acts as a catalyst or lubricant to the process of change.

THE IMPORTANCE OF INTERMEDIATE GOALS

> We must be prepared to work with those who continue to misuse drugs to help them reduce the risks involved in doing so, above all the risk of acquiring or spreading HIV. Reaching this less well motivated group will necessitate a more proactive approach and a readiness to work initially towards goals which fall short of abstinence . . . there are however no 'master strokes' which will deliver the achievement of these goals . . . the greatest benefit is more likely to accrue from the sum of multiple small gains deriving from an integrated and responsive strategy than from any single approach.
>
> (Advisory Council on the Misuse of Drugs 1988: 17–18)

As soon as the special problems presented by HIV are taken on board, it becomes clear that there is special benefit that would be accrued by the individual and by society from specific changes in drug-taking behaviour. Thus, the cessation of sharing of injecting equipment and more generally the move from injectable to oral drug use become highly significant steps forward, even though dependence on the drug might continue. By identifying these subgoals or intermediate goals, it becomes possible to work towards (and measure progress towards) certain key points in the journey of treatment.

For each individual patient, the prescribing options should be gauged according to the extent to which they may promote flow through one or more processes of change. Intermediate goals might be the move from sharing to non-sharing, from injectible to oral drug use, or the stabilisation of formerly chaotic drug use, for example. The simple model of process of change needs to be adapted to accommodate intermediate goals. An overall treatment plan might thus be seen as comprising a *cascade* of processes of change with each 'maintenance' state being an intermediate goal (see Figure 19.2).

Treatment might be expected to promote flow through the cascade of processes of change with particular emphasis being placed on one or other element of flow at each point in the total treatment plan. The intermediate goals (and their respective processes of change) may be dealt with sequentially or simultaneously, but it is important to acknowledge the particular benefit of some intermediate goals and also to monitor the potential retrograde flow that may occur with other goals.

Figure 19.2 Cascade of processes of change

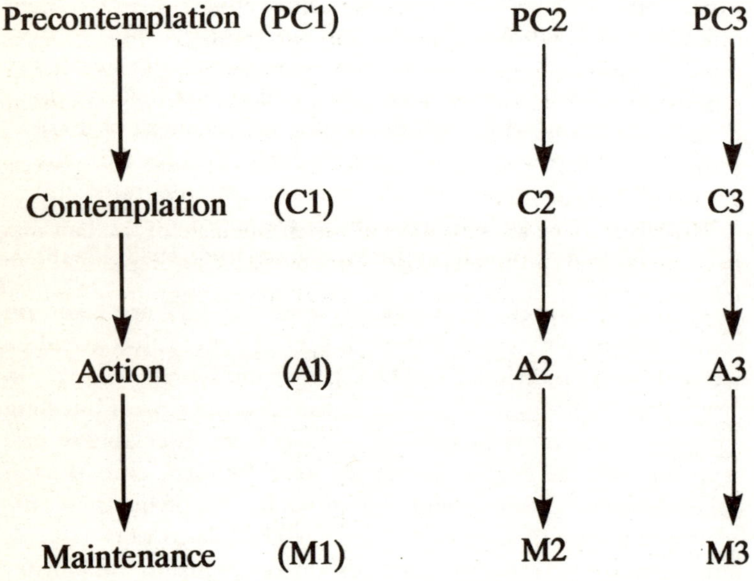

CAPTURE, RETENTION AND THROUGHPUT

If the bus route is to be effective, then it must capture a good number of travellers, it must operate in such a way that they are held voluntarily 'captive' for a sufficient length of time; and it must ensure that this time is used productively so that at the end of this period they are at another place (their treatment destination) and not just merely older but otherwise unmoved.

Capture

Capture depends in large part on a willingness to be caught, although coercive pressures (such as from family or the courts) may help latent motivation to become manifest. Various types of prescribing may act as capture 'bait' and these have been considered in more detail in Chapter 13. To be effective, bait must attract. There are different types of bait, not all of which involve prescribing. The offer of assistance with benefits and welfare rights may attract, as may the offer of legal aid. A drug worker makes a daily visit to the police cells to recruit for a methadone programme; or a project may negotiate with the courts for a drug offender to attend a programme for assessment and planning of rehabilitation options. The recently established syringe-exchange schemes constitute another example in which a bait other than the drugs themselves is employed, and it is probable that the harm-reduction advice and general health care may add to the general appeal of these services.

However, there are also ways in which the taste of the bait may become tainted. If the response is not available at time of need or there are too many visible conditions attached, then the potential appeal of the bait may not be realised. It is crucially important to understand that the measure of the effectiveness of the bait is *not* the degree of uptake of the bait itself, but is the extent of progress on to the next stage. Drug services which allow easy referral from voluntary agencies, casualty departments, the police and courts and self-referral are likely to attract a wider variety of drug users; whereas if the service is run in such a way that it only recognises gross indicators of drug use then it may fail to identify less problematic drug users who may be at an earlier stage in their drug-using career and might be helped by simpler interventions.

Retention

All drug services appear beset with problems of poor retention. There is a widespread problem of decay of the captured population over the first few appointments, and this phenomenon appears to extend across a range of types of service, including out-patient prescribing programmes, drug-free therapeutic communities and syringe exchange schemes. In the new HIV-conscious climate, it is necessary to look for ways of increasing the 'stickiness' of the service, so that once drug users make contact with the service there is a greater likelihood that they will remain in contact and thus continue to be available for secondary preventive and treatment approaches to be applied. Might prescribing be effective for some of these patients as an adhesive which increases the 'stickiness' of the service? This debate has become more relevant with the growing interest in harm-reduction approaches and the identification of intermediate goals, and there is now a need to look afresh at drug treatment services to see whether there is evidence that they might increase the likelihood of achieving such intermediate goals as the cessation of injectible drug use. It is already possible to identify features which appear to reduce the 'stickiness' of the service – features such as long waiting lists, delay for appointments, an unfriendly environment and a stigmatising service, all of which appear to reduce the likelihood that the drug user will attend subsequent appointments. It may be possible to introduce positive reinforcers which increase the likelihood of subsequent reattendance. Quite apart from the removal of obstacles, reattendance rates may improve with the provision of assistance with housing, employment, and the provision of recreational activities and legal aid as well as direct drug services. Contingent provision of some of these facilities is now being incorporated into a few treatment programmes in the UK, but data are not yet available on their effectiveness as possible enhancers of compliance.

Throughput

Throughput is a component which is often omitted from consideration in analyses of drug treatment services. This is surprising, for without evidence of change in the behaviour in the drug user it is difficult to see what purpose has been served by the service. If change is a *sine qua non* of treatment, then how can the effectiveness of a service be gauged without some prior identification of the goals of the service? Without adequate consideration of throughput and with the constraints of finite resources, there is a danger that the service might silt up. Such a sorry state of affairs existed in London drug clinics in the early 1980s, at which time new treatment slots were virtually unavailable at the NHS drug clinics as they were already occupied by long-term opiate addicts, some of whom had been in receipt of their prescriptions on an uninterrupted basis for well over a decade. Quite apart from the debate that has occurred as to whether or not such maintenance prescribing was a legitimate form of treatment in such services, there can be no doubt that the circumstances were unacceptable. There existed a treatment 'apartheid', with the privilege of treatment availability being reserved for those who had entered treatment during the early years of the clinics while the unfortunate latecomers were denied any more than the most cursory of services.

PROMOTING FLOW THROUGH THE PROCESS OF CHANGE

The guiding principles which have been put forward by the Advisory Council on the Misuse of Drugs (1989) for assessing the appropriateness of prescribing also serve to emphasise the importance of flow through the process of change and hence progress through treatment. In Part II of their report on *AIDS and Drug Misuse* (1989) the ACMD identify four criteria which have a bearing on the decision whether or not to prescribe to the drug taker:

> We see no reason to depart from the principle that prescribing should never be undertaken without an identified goal. However, if a drug misuser is known to be seropositive, a wider range of goals should be considered, including the following:
> (a) to attract seropositive drug misusers into regular contact with services;
> (b) to promote behaviour change away from practices which carry a risk of transmitting HIV infection;

> (c) to promote behaviour change in such a way as to maximise personal health and stability;
> (d) to encourage compliance with medical treatment, including regular check ups, and the regular self-administration of antiviral drugs such as zidovudine [AZT].
>
> The first of these goals is not an end in itself, but rather the platform on which the others are founded.
>
> (ACMD, 1989)

As they point out, criterion (a) is not sufficient in itself but describes the context within which criteria (b), (c) and/or (d) might be seen to exist.

Thus, it might be appropriate for treatment services to be more tolerant of lapses or hiccups that occur in the hoped-for smooth course of treatment, provided there is evidence that beneficial change might still accrue. Edwards (1982) has described the basic work of treatment as 'nudging down natural pathways of recovery'. Treatment should do more than just mark time while awaiting some presumed natural maturing-out process; it should hasten the arrival of identified beneficial changes.

Should there be special treatment programmes for HIV-positive drug users with preferential access to treatment and possibly with access to forms of treatment that would not be available to the broader drug-using population? The ACMD considered these suggestions and concluded that such a system was unworkable and inappropriate; they recommended that the correct strategy was to increase the availability (nature of service, speed of response, convenience of locality, etc.) for the whole drug-using population – irrespective of presumed or actual HIV status. Thus, the HIV-positive drug user should be dealt with in the context of an integrated system of health care rather than receiving a service through segregation from the broader drug-taking population. The criteria which should be borne in mind in deciding on treatment responses have been described above. It will be seen that these criteria should be applied equally across the broader drug-taking population, even though there may be certain circumstances in which HIV illness or asymptomatic seropositivity might lead to the identification of goals that would otherwise not have been considered.

If drug treatment services are to improve their capacities for capture, retention and throughput, then they will need to allow prescribing to return to a more central position in their work and to recognise the considerable benefit that may result from the achievement of key intermediate goals.

CONCLUSION

Change is what treatment is all about. The worth of treatment A or B for a particular drug taker can be gauged according to the extent to which it successfully enables the achievement of key 'intermediate goals'. Absolute reliance on treatment A or B (or any other single treatment) should be avoided as it will reduce the potential of the service to fulfil the functions of capture, retention and throughput for as large and as wide a drug-using population as possible. By recognising the special value of certain intermediate goals, it should be possible to provide a wider range of treatment plans which are more closely suited to the particular circumstances of the individual drug taker, whilst still promoting movement by that individual through a cascade of processes of change.

REFERENCES

Advisory Council on the Misuse of Drugs (1988) *AIDS and Drug Misuse Report: Part I*, London: HMSO.

Advisory Council on the Misuse of Drugs (1989) *AIDS and Drug Misuse Report: Part II*, London: HMSO.

Edwards, G. (1982) *The Treatment of Drinking Problems: A Guide for the Helping Professions*, London: Grant McIntyre.

Presidential Commission on the Human Immunodeficiency Virus Epidemic (1988) *Report*, Washington.

Prochaska, J.O. and Di Clemente, C.O. (1986) 'Toward a comprehensive model of change', in: W.R. Miller and N. Heather (eds) *Treating Addictive Behaviours: Processes of Change*, New York and London: Plenum Press.

Chapter Twenty

DISTRIBUTING STERILE NEEDLES AND SYRINGES TO PEOPLE WHO INJECT DRUGS: THE SYRINGE-EXCHANGE EXPERIMENT

GERRY V. STIMSON, MARTIN C. DONOGHOE, RACHEL LART AND KATE DOLAN

The idea of giving syringes to people who inject drugs strikes many as a strange way to try to prevent drug problems. For many years it was argued that the availability of syringes was an important factor encouraging the spread of drug problems, and policies were pursued to restrict their use.

In many states in the USA with a high prevalence of injectors, 'drug paraphernalia' laws limit availability and possession of syringes by drug users, or require prescriptions for their sale and possession (Pascal 1988).

Swedish laws against 'facilitating drug abuse' prevent the sale of syringes to addicts, and Sweden is the only country in Europe where needles and syringes cannot be purchased in pharmacies.

In New South Wales, Australia, it was until 1986 a criminal offence to carry equipment for the purpose of injecting drugs (Wolk *et al.* 1988).

In Scotland, the common-law offence of 'reckless conduct' once acted as a deterrent to potential suppliers.

In the UK, the pharmacists' professional association advised members against selling syringes to drug users, on the grounds that to do so would increase the prevalence of injecting drug use.

Now, however, many countries are making syringes available to injectors, or have seriously considered doing so. What has forced this change?

Like many other aspects of our drug and social policies, the need to prevent the spread of HIV has brought a radical rethinking of policy. Despite concerns about 'condoning' drug use, a more pragmatic public health position has emerged in some countries. In essence, the reasoning is that HIV and AIDS are more of a threat to individual and public health than drug use; that there will be many people who are currently injecting and who are unable or unwilling to stop; and that something must be done to reduce both their risk of HIV infection, and that of transmission to others. Giving sterile needles and syringes may be one way to reduce the spread of HIV – this was one of the conclusions reached at a significant World Health Organization meeting in late 1986 (World Health Organization, 1986).

THE RATIONALE FOR SYRINGE DISTRIBUTION

The theory is relatively simple. HIV can be spread through blood products, and sharing syringes is an effective way to pass blood from one person to another. People who inject drugs are likely to share syringes. In Edinburgh, 63 per cent of patients attending an HIV screening clinic reported sharing syringes at least once a week (Brettle 1986). In Melbourne, Australia, 91 per cent of injectors had shared at some time (Paine *et al.* 1985). In surveys conducted in England, Wales and Scotland, 62 per cent had shared in the last four weeks, with higher rates in Scotland (76 per cent) and among injectors not in touch with services (Stimson *et al.* 1988a).

These levels of syringe sharing have serious implications for the potential transmission of HIV. In a survey of syringe-exchange clients, 27 per cent used a syringe that had already been used by someone else an average of 12 times in the last four weeks. If this behaviour is typical of other people who inject drugs, and assuming that there are 60,000 injectors in the UK, there would be 2.5 million occasions annually when injectors are at risk of acquiring HIV. In fact, this is an underestimate: syringe-exchange clients have lower rates of sharing than other injectors.

Why do injectors share syringes?

There are many reasons why people share syringes. These include a dislike of carrying them (especially where there are laws against syringe possession or where they may be used by police as evidence of drug possession), social situations between friends where sharing drugs and syringes is *de rigueur*, sharing with sexual partners who are perceived as being 'safe', and in circumstances where syringes are unavailable (for example, late at night, when buying drugs, or when in prison).

The most common reason is difficulty in obtaining syringes. In Melbourne this was reported by 66 per cent (Paine *et al.* 1985). In the UK surveys it was reported by between 44 per cent and 56 per cent (Stimson *et al.* 1988a). Lack of availability was commonly cited even in Italy, where needles and syringes are sold in pharmacies – injectors said that there were difficulties in obtaining syringes, especially at the time they were needed (Martin *et al.* 1988). Many observers consider that official pressure to restrict supplies of syringes was a significant factor in the rapid spread of HIV in Edinburgh (see Chapter 9).

Providing the knowledge and the means to change

Any strategy that reduces the level of sharing should be of considerable help in preventing the spread of HIV. The evidence that some injectors share because syringes are hard to obtain suggests the potential benefit from increasing availability.

The strategy is based on a *knowledge* and *means* approach to enabling behavioural change. People are provided with information about the changes that need to be made, and with the means to change – sterile needles and syringes (and condoms).

DELIVERING SYRINGES TO INJECTORS

Syringes have been supplied in a number of ways, the main differences being the method of delivery (e.g. the agency responsible for supply), the type of staff involved, whether there are other services on offer, how the service is funded, and whether syringes must be returned.

Supply only

In a few exceptional circumstances syringes have been supplied from vending machines (in Bremen and Copenhagen). The service is anonymous, requires few staff (except to fill machines) and is available around the clock. There are a number of problems, including restricting sale to bona fide injectors, and getting syringes returned. This latter problem has been solved with a new machine which accepts used syringes, and will soon be in use in Spain as well as Denmark. The biggest disadvantage to drug services (but not necessarily to injectors) is the limited opportunities for making contacts with customers and offering advice and other help.

In some countries needles and syringes are available from pharmacies. In Italy and Spain they are available without restriction from pharmacies; in Austria they have been available since 1985 (Fuchs *et al.* 1988), and in France since 1987 (Espinoza *et al.* 1988).

But in some countries, even where it is legal to sell syringes, some pharmacists are reluctant to do so because of the undesirability of having injectors on the premises. In Glasgow only one in five pharmacists was willing to sell syringes (Kohli and Goldberg 1988). In parts of Britain, Australia and France there have been special attempts to involve pharmacists. In one UK scheme they are paid to participate, provided with facilities for the disposal of used syringes, offered advice and referral channels for clients in need of other help, and participating pharmacists are identified by a special sign. In New South Wales, Australia, a pharmacy project took four months to establish, operates at low cost, covers 40 per cent of the state, and 500,000 syringes were distributed in 1987 (Phua *et al.* 1988).

Syringe exchange: supply and return of equipment

The distinctive feature of syringe exchange is that needles and syringes are given to injectors on an *exchange* basis. One reason is a public health concern that used and possibly infected needles should not be left in public places, or disposed of in a way that may be hazardous to others. Exchanging syringes also reduces the likelihood that they will be circulated and reused. Syringes can be distributed with satisfactory rates of return – 70 per cent in Amsterdam in 1987, rising to 95 per cent in 1988 (Buning *et al.* 1988), around 62 per cent in the UK (Stimson *et al.* 1988b), and 41 per cent in New South Wales (Wolk *et al.* 1988). The fact that the client must return to the agency increases the opportunity for advice and counselling.

In Holland syringe distribution was started by the *junkiebond* (the union of drug users) in 1984 in response to the hepatitis B epidemic and is now conducted by a variety of agencies, usually ancillary to their other activities. For example, many low-threshold methadone clinics, including the 'methadone bus', make syringes (and condoms) available, and have facilities for their return. In 1987, 700,000 syringes were distributed at 11 locations in Amsterdam (see Chapter 14).

SYRINGE EXCHANGE IN THE UK

Some syringe exchanges were running in the UK in 1986. A major impetus came in a government-sponsored experiment in 1987–8, where 15 agencies in England and Scotland collaborated in a pilot project (Stimson *et al.* 1988b). The number of syringe-exchange schemes grew to around 120 by the end of 1989.

Some agencies added syringe exchange on to their existing work. In others, the syringe exchange is a special agency – for example, a shopfront, a caravan, or an office in a drug agency or on a medical site. In addition to syringes and condoms, most offer counselling about HIV, sexual behaviour, and drug problems; some offer primary medical and social care and the possibility of referral to other helping agencies.

A key feature is that the schemes claim to be 'user friendly' — that is, psychologically and physically accessible, with low thresholds for eligibility, minimal identification, and informal relationships with clients. Most of the agencies in the UK pilot project saw their aims and philosophy centred on both HIV prevention (risk reduction) and harm minimisation (i.e. minimising a wide range of health and social risks associated with injecting drugs).

EVIDENCE FOR EFFECTIVENESS

The ultimate criterion of success is the impact on the spread of HIV among clients and among injectors in communities with syringe exchanges. There is no conclusive research evidence to show that this is the case, due in part to the short time-scale over which syringe exchanges have been evaluated. There is some suggestive evidence of sustained low rates of HIV from a syringe exchange in Sydney, where returned syringes have been examined for the presence of HIV antibodies (Wolk *et al.* 1988; Wodak *et al.* 1988).

Initially, effectiveness has been judged by whether syringe exchange has reached target recipients and is operating successfully, and whether people who attend report changes in their behaviour.

In the UK, syringe exchanges have reached considerable numbers of injectors. Many clients are not in touch with other services and have had little former help for drug problems. The clients tend to be opiate users, but there are also some primary amphetamine injectors, which is significant in the UK context because these people are rarely attracted to formal treatment services. They tend to be older, longer-term injectors, and women are underrepresented.

One surprising finding is a high turnover of clients. When syringe exchange first started it was thought that clients would enrol and become regular customers. The reasons why this did not happen include a combination of positive outcomes (referral to treatment, cessation of injecting) and negative ones (continued injection without a regular supply of clean equipment, imprisonment, death); and the fact that the schemes are not a cartel – there are other suppliers.

What about clients' risk behaviour? Syringe-exchange clients report lower initial risk behaviour than other injectors. At intake about 35 per cent say they have recently shared, compared with the rates around 60 per cent reported in other studies. Many who continued to attend reported an improvement in behaviour, so that in three months of attendance the basic rate of sharing was reduced to 27 per cent. In other words, 73 per cent were not sharing, to which can be added a further 6 per cent who continued to share, but at a reduced level. Overall, a total of 79 per cent of continuing attenders sustained low risk injecting behaviour, adopted low-risk behaviour, or reduced their level of risk behaviour. The rate of sharing is now amongst the lowest recorded in the UK literature. There were also other desirable changes, such as a reduction in the range of drugs used and injected, and in the frequency of injecting.

Staff reported difficulty in discussing sexual behaviour with clients. Nevertheless, changes in sexual behaviour included a reduction in the number of sexual partners. The only increase in risk behaviour was a decrease in condom use.

In Amsterdam, the syringe exchanges have been assessed by a study which compared people who use the exchanges frequently (exchangers) and those who don't (non-exchangers). The exchangers exposed themselves less often to high-risk situations, and had lower rates of sharing (Buning *et al.* 1988).

The results support the argument that drug injectors can be helped to make changes in their behaviour which could be of cumulative importance in reducing the spread of HIV. Whether these changes are sufficient in magnitude and durability to have this impact remains to be seen.

There is still a lot that needs to be investigated. Nothing is known about the impact on the prevalence of injecting, and the UK lacks baseline and longitudinal data which would enable such an assessment to be made. Likewise, nothing is known about impact on demand for treatment, because there are no comprehensive data on the numbers of drug users treated by drug services. However, there is evidence that in Amsterdam the prevalence of injecting has not increased, and that the demand for methadone treatment has continued to increase (see Chapter 14). Assessment of potential negative effects of social policies is methodologically difficult, but there is clearly more work to be done.

OBSTACLES AND FUTURE DEVELOPMENTS

Syringe exchange remains a controversial approach in many countries. In Sweden, there has been a small experiment in Lund, and despite possible legal problems the authorities have not interfered (Ljundberg *et al.* 1988; Des Jarlais and Woods 1988). In Switzerland, availability varies from canton to canton – in Berne, syringes are provided free of charge, while in other cantons they are completely banned (World Health Organization, 1986). Various groups trying to establish schemes in the USA have faced legal and political obstacles, with objections from both white and black politicians, and a political directive prevents the National Institute on Drug Abuse from funding projects or research on syringe exchange. In November 1988 a limited experiment with 200 clients started in New York City. The extreme caution found in the

USA has placed the burden of evidence on countries with fewer research resources.

What are the limits to syringe exchange?

First, certain limits relate to the clients: despite improvements in the availability of clean needles and syringes in the UK, a minority continued to engage in high-risk behaviours, suggesting that there are further obstacles to individual risk reduction. The syringe-exchange prevention strategy, based on a *knowledge* and *means* approach inadequately considers other factors that make it difficult for people to change their behaviour. Exhorting injectors to change their behaviour, and providing syringes, does not address a central problem: many people find it difficult to adopt safer behaviour. The circumstances in which drug use and sexual behaviour occur may inhibit the adoption of safer practices. Prevention strategies need to address the factors that make it difficult for injectors to adopt and sustain safe behaviour.

Second, certain limits derive from the service itself: syringe exchanges do not reach some groups of injectors. In the UK they need to reach a greater number of younger injectors with a shorter history of injecting, and more women. It is also clear that injectors who are not reached are at higher risk than people who come to syringe exchange. Many are unwilling to come to office-based programmes, and other approaches such as outreach may be required.

Third, now that it has been demonstrated that the service can operate successfully, syringe exchange workers must develop the service and its effectiveness. With a high client turnover, syringe exchanges need to maximise the impact of one-off contacts, to improve their ability to maintain contact, and to examine the potential for referral to other help. There is also a need to develop counselling, advice and information techniques, since our assessment is that agency staff have yet to develop efficacious ways of helping people to change.

CONCLUSION

When needle and syringe exchange was first introduced, some people thought that it would be the major single, simple solution that would make it possible for recalcitrant injectors to change their behaviour. It should not surprise those familiar with prevention and treatment research to learn that this is not so. Many forms of help and treatment for drug users achieve only modest short-term benefits, although the longer-term outcome is more optimistic.

Syringe exchange is still a novel measure and, compared with the experience and research evidence gained with other approaches (for example, methadone maintenance), it is still in its infancy. The evidence so far is that syringe exchange reaches injectors who are not in touch with other services, that it does this at reasonable cost, is delivered in a way that is acceptable to most clients, helps some drug injectors maintain low-risk behaviours, and helps some others to adopt them. It has areas that need to be developed, which is only to be expected in any innovative service, and it does not reach all drug injectors. It has considerable potential as a low-threshold contact for drug injectors within an overall preventive and helping response.

REFERENCES

Brettle, R.P. (1986) 'Epidemic of AIDS related virus infection among intravenous drug abusers', *British Medical Journal* 292: 1671.

Buning, E.C., Hartgers, T., Verster, A., van Santen, G.W. and Coutinho, R.A. (1988) 'Needle and syringe exchange in Amsterdam', poster presented at the 4th International Conference on AIDS, Stockholm.

Des Jarlais, D.C. and Woods, J.S. (1988) 'Needle exchanges', *Newsletter: International Working Group on AIDS and IV Drug Use* 3(1): 1.

Espinoza, P., Bouchard, I., Ballian J., and Devoto, P. (1988), 'Has the open sale of syringes modified the syringe exchanging habits of drug addicts?', poster presented at the 4th International Conference on AIDS, Stockholm.

Fuchs, D., Unterweger, B., Hausen. A. *et al.* (1988) 'Anti-HIV antibodies, anti-HTLV-1 antibodies and neopterin levels in parenteral drug addicts in the Austrian Tyrol', *Journal of Acquired Immune Deficiency Syndromes* 1: 65.

Kohli, H.S. and Goldberg D.J. (1988) 'Intravenous drug misuse: has the pharmacist a role?', *Health Bulletin* 46(2): 122.

Ljundberg, B., Andersson, B., Christensson, B., Hugo-Persson, M., Tunving K. and Ursing, B. (1988) 'Distribution of sterile equipment to IV drug abusers as part of an HIV intervention program', poster presented at the 4th International Conference on AIDS, Stockholm.

Martin, G.S., Serpelloni, G., Galvan U., Rizzetto, A. and Gomma M. (1988) 'Results obtained from an AIDS education intervention aimed at raising the informational level of IVDAs', Verona: mimeo.
Paine, S., Tonuma, M. and Monhelt, B. (1985) 'AIDS in drug abusers', *Medical Journal of Australia* 143: 631.
Pascal, C.B. (1988) 'Intravenous drug abuse and AIDS transmission: federal and state laws regulating needle availability', in R.J. Battjes and R.W. Pickens (eds) *Needle Sharing among Intravenous Drug Abusers: National and International Perspectives,* Washington: National Institute on Drug Abuse, Monograph Series 80.
Phua, R., Goh, T., Webeck, P. and Mullins J. (1988) 'The control and spread of HIV infection among IV drug users in NSW, Australia: Evaluation of the needle and syringes distribution program through retail pharmacies – NSW 1987', poster presented at 1st International Conference on the Global Impact of AIDS, London.
Stimson, G.V., Alldritt, L., Dolan, K., Donoghoe, M. and Lart R.A. (1988a) *Injecting Equipment Exchange Schemes: Final Report,* London: Goldsmiths' College.
Stimson, G.V., Alldritt, L., Dolan, K. and Donoghoe, M. (1988b) 'Syringe exchange schemes for drug users in England and Scotland', *British Medical Journal* 296: 1717.
Wodak, A., Dolan, K., Imrie, A.I. *et al.* (1988) 'Antibodies to the Human Immunodeficiency Virus in needles and syringes used by intravenous drug abusers', *Medical Journal of Australia* 147: 275.
Wolk, J., Wodak, A., Morlet, A. *et al.* (1988) 'Syringe HIV seroprevalence and behavioural and demographic characteristics of intravenous drug users in Sydney, Australia, 1987', *AIDS* 2(5): 373.
World Health Organization (1986) *Consultation on AIDS among Drug Abusers,* Stockholm: World Health Organization Regional Office for Europe.

Chapter Twenty-one

COUNSELLING THE DRUG TAKER ABOUT HIV INFECTION AND AIDS

JOHN GREEN

The counselling of those affected by HIV infection and AIDS has been recognised as a major part of helping them almost since the beginning of the AIDS epidemic. However, most of the published work in the area relates to the counselling of gay men or haemophiliacs. With few exceptions (e.g. Mulleady 1988) little has been published on the details of how to counsel drug users about HIV, except in terms of specific infection-control advice. There is a sizeable volume of published work detailing the best ways to set up services, to sterilise syringes or needles or to spread health education material, but much less on how to help users to reduce their risks in face-to-face discussion or how to promote psychological well-being in the HIV-positive drug users.

This chapter briefly surveys some of the general issues in counselling which apply to all those affected by HIV infection and tries to pick out those issues which are different for drug users and other individuals at risk from HIV. It is also valuable to look at the more extensive experience of HIV counselling with homosexuals and to consider areas of similarity and dissimilarity.

PURPOSES OF COUNSELLING IN HIV AND AIDS

The following sections discuss the two key aims of counselling in HIV/AIDS.

The prevention of the spread of infection

In general, *the same changes which prevent an individual infected with HIV passing it on also prevent someone not yet infected acquiring the infection* (Green 1989). So someone who always uses a condom in sex will not, if they use them carefully and avoid breakages, acquire HIV infection sexually. Nor, if they are already infected, will they pass it on to a partner. The same principle applies to syringe sharing. The importance of this consideration is considerable. Many workers still see the HIV test as being a *sine qua non* of successful counselling – it is clearly not. It is possible – indeed, essential – to provide successful counselling to all those at risk, i.e. to seropositives, seronegatives and those who have not been tested.

Maximisation of psychological and social well-being

When counselling services are set up for those with HIV/AIDS it is the prevention of spread of infection which tends to attract most interest, at least from funding bodies. However, it is important to note that those who have AIDS or who are infected with HIV often experience a great deal of distress and disruption to their lives. One of the key aims of counselling is to reduce this distress and there is evidence that this is achievable. Even if counselling did not make any impact whatsoever on behaviour, it would still be important in reducing distress and helping those affected by the virus to maximise their quality of life.

The above two aims refer chiefly to those who are at risk or who are infected. However, it is important to note that HIV often affects a wider range of people and these too will need help and counselling. The families of those who are infected, their lovers, wives, husbands, informal carers – all need support and help. Indeed, in some cases they may need more support and help than the person infected with HIV.

BASIC PRINCIPLES

Counselling should be a dialogue in which the counsellor and the client work together. The counsellor needs to listen to the difficulties which the client has before seeking to offer advice. Although this seems an obvious point, it is all too often honoured in the breach rather than the observance.

Counselling is vital for the drug taker, irrespective of whether the person chooses to be tested or not. HIV counselling should not be seen as merely relevant for those who choose to be tested –

indeed, it could be argued that it is just as relevant or even more relevant for those who choose not to be tested. It is important that clients understand the risks associated with certain aspects of their drug-taking and sexual behaviour and recognise the changes in behaviour that will reduce or remove these risks; and the decision not to be tested or a negative test result must not be seen as reasons why the at-risk behaviour can continue.

Advice which is offered also has to be practical. Advice on sterilisation of syringes and needles which suggests elaborate procedures is not likely to be adopted if it is simply impracticable in terms of the client's way of using drugs. Advice to use a clean syringe will not be taken up if clean syringes are not readily available. Help and advice need to be offered in a way which fits in with the behaviour of the client. Only by finding out in detail about the life-style of the client is it possible to help make positive changes.

Probably nowhere is this issue more obvious than in terms of sexual behaviour. It is easy to advise people always to use a condom. However, they have to be able to obtain condoms, to afford them if they are not free. They have to be able to persuade a partner to use or allow them to use a condom. This may require some degree of negotiating skills. They may have to make quite large changes in the way that they go about their sexual lives in order to put 'safer sex' into practice. A lot of people have sex with a new partner when they are drunk or under the influence of drugs. These are conditions under which they are least likely to be thinking about protecting themselves and their partner. In order to put safer sex into their lives, they may have to think ahead and plan their sex lives much more than they have done in the past.

The most effective counselling takes place when both the counsellor and the client work together to achieve agreed goals and where they aim to generate practical solutions to practical problems.

There is no way in which a counsellor can force people to change their behaviour. Good counselling involves joint problem-solving between the client, who has the problem, and the counsellor, who should have information and who is at least partially detached from the problem. It is vitally important to lead the client to come up with his or her own solutions to staying well. Solutions imposed by arousing fear ('If you don't do this you will die . . .') or by force of personality ('I'm the expert, do what I say . . .') are doomed to be effective only in the short term, if at all.

A particular problem with drug users is the difficulty of engaging them in the counselling process. A sizeable proportion of users are erratic attenders. Even so, it is possible to engage users in counselling, provided the counsellor is seen to address those issues which are relevant to the users themselves. Rather than being a process in which counsellors go through their own agenda, counselling *must* be relevant to the counselled.

Good counselling skills alone are not sufficient for someone to be able to counsel effectively about HIV/AIDS. It is necessary to have a good background knowledge of the facts about HIV. Since the information available keeps changing, particularly with respect to new therapies and approaches to treatment, it is essential that anyone working in the area keep closely in touch with the scientific literature in the field.

FINDING OUT ABOUT THE CLIENT

Getting a good picture of the client's life and the roots of risk behaviours is essential but is also difficult. In order to help people to modify their risk behaviour it is necessary to find out what the behaviour is. This means asking very specific, very clear questions. There is no doubt that many counsellors find this difficult to do. They will often not ask important questions because of their fear that the client will be offended, particularly where those questions are about sex or use of illicit drugs. However, clients are rarely offended by these questions if these seem appropriate – which, in the context of HIV, they usually are.

In counselling people about HIV/AIDS it is important to get clear information about their sexual behaviour. It is important to find out what they do sexually – do they have vaginal sex, oral sex, anal sex? What other sexual behaviours do they engage in? Who do they have sex with? Do they have sex only with a regular partner, or with casual partners, or both? What does sex mean to them? Is it a means of release, or do they engage in it for excitement or because it provides closeness to another person or because they get paid for it? Is there a difference in their sexual behaviour and what they get out of sex with casual partners as opposed to a regular partner? What contraceptive precautions do they take?

How acceptable are condoms or other means of reducing risk to them and to their partners (Green 1988a)?

Similar considerations apply to helping someone to modify their injecting behaviour. It is important to find out about sharing of syringes, why they share, whether they understand the risks, whether they have access to clean syringes, whether they sterilise their syringes and, if so, how often and how effectively. It is also important to ascertain how acceptable other ways of taking drugs, such as orally or by inhalation, would be (Mulleady 1988). It is necessary to look beyond just the presence or absence of sharing of injecting equipment and to examine the frequency of such risk-taking behaviour – in what contexts does it occur? With which particular people are they sharing? What significance does injecting hold for the individual?

The key elements are to find out what behaviours people engage in and why they engage in those behaviours. Without knowing what motivates people to do particular things it is very difficult to help them to change them.

Finding out about the client also means finding out about other aspects of their lives, their social lives, their housing, their relationships and their hopes for the future or lack of hopes. Where counselling goes wrong, it often does so because of lack of understanding of the client's life rather than lack of technique on the part of the counsellor.

GENERAL APPROACHES TO HIV/AIDS COUNSELLING

Good counselling skills may not always come naturally but they can be learnt. Different workers have approached the problems presented by HIV/AIDS counselling in different ways and from different starting-points. Some workers have adopted a cognitive approach (Green 1986; Green and McCreaner 1988; Miller 1987). Other workers have adopted a systems approach (Miller and Bor 1988). Others still have adopted psychodynamic (Namir 1986), co-counselling or humanistic approaches.

What is it that successful approaches have in common? They help the client to come up with changes they can make in their lives and help them to make those changes. There is a common core in the approaches which all workers have used which is specific to HIV/AIDS. Beyond that common core the specific approach to be used is likely to depend on the way in which the worker has been trained and the working style in which he or she feels most comfortable.

THE STRUCTURE OF COUNSELLING

Counselling those at risk

There is little point in waiting until people are infected before counselling them. The first priority of any counselling service aimed at drug users must be to provide counselling about HIV/AIDS to all users who are at risk.

This should be relatively easy with users who are attending for treatment for drug dependence. However, only a minority of users in an area are likely to be receiving treatment at any given moment. Within the medical services in an area, other workers are also likely to be in contact with drug users and in a position to offer counselling to them or to refer them on. General practitioners, general medical staff, family planning staff, health visitors and a range of other community and hospital staff are likely to be in contact with drug users. It is important to provide appropriate training to them to allow them to carry out the work or to provide ready access to counselling for their clients.

Counselling with drug users, a largely heterosexual group, needs to cover not just the issues surrounding sex and syringes but also the key area of pregnancy. Not just female drug users but also the sexual partners of male drug users may become infected with HIV and pass it on to their unborn child. The rate of transmission from mother to foetus is high – probably between 20 and 50 per cent, depending on the health of the mother. If the mother is symptomatic there is a theoretical risk that the pregnancy may hasten the progress of HIV disease in the mother, although studies supporting or refuting this are not yet available (Schoenbaum *et al.* 1988). It is important at this moment that every young woman who is at risk, and every man who is putting his partner at risk, should understand these issues, have access to good contraceptive advice and the wherewithal, and understand the need to seek further advice as soon as they suspect a pregnancy.

PRE-TEST COUNSELLING

In most developed countries and in an increasing number of developing countries, the intention is that HIV testing should be available on demand. However, whether it is helpful for an individual to have an HIV test is likely to vary with personal circumstances. The considerable distress which being tested for HIV created in individuals when the HIV test was first made available highlighted the key importance of pre-test counselling for all those contemplating the test.

It is believed by some workers that having the test in itself encourages individuals to change their risk behaviours. In fact, the reality is much more complex. In 1987 a meeting called by the US Centers for Disease Control (CDC) reviewed the evidence and concluded that 'The self knowledge or awareness of their HIV antibody status apparently had only a minor influence on behavior change on the part of those persons who self-identify as being at risk of HIV infection and AIDS.' This illustrates how difficult it is to reach clear conclusions which have direct relevance to the continuation, cessation or modification of risk behaviours and the way in which HIV testing might have an influence on these behaviours.

It is important to remember that, for most individuals at risk, the changes in behaviour which will prevent them from becoming infected if they are not already infected are the same changes which will prevent them from infecting others if they are already infected.

Some individuals want to have the test because they feel that it will help them personally to change; others because they 'would rather know'. These reasons are good reasons for being tested. In the case of the woman who has been at risk and wishes to know her status before becoming pregnant, or the pregnant woman who would prefer termination to the risk of having an infected baby, there are strong reasons for being tested.

Against any possible advantage of the test must be set the distress to individuals of finding that they are positive, the social discrimination if they choose to tell others and the fact that there is nothing currently that can be offered in the way of treatment for an asymptomatic seropositive.

It is important that anyone contemplating the HIV test should be able to go through the issues in detail and to reach a personal decision about what is best for them. They need to be prepared for the different possible results. They need to understand the meaning of the test – expecting drug users to take in the implications of being infected when they have just been given a positive test result is simply unreasonable. Good pre-test counselling must be a priority wherever the test is offered. McCreaner (1988, 1989) has given good accounts of the issues and approach.

POST-TEST COUNSELLING

Regardless of whether an individual has a positive or negative test result (or remains untested), he or she should be counselled. The individual who finds himself or herself positive will often find the result devastating. Careful support and help will be needed during the period of adjusting to the result. Not only is there the issue of being infected with a virus which may at some future time cause them to become ill and die but, if they have not already done so, such individuals are also faced with making changes in their lives to avoid the transmission of the virus to others and to avoid acquiring other infections sexually or through syringe sharing which may impair their health and possibly hasten progression to AIDS.

Appropriate counselling involves more than just supporting and guiding through the necessary changes in life-style; it means helping the individual to come to terms with the change in self-image and expectations which is associated with being positive. Counselling for someone who is seropositive can only be set in the context of a comprehensive approach to care. Help with drug usage – whether help to come off, to change from injecting to other routes of drug usage or to alter the risk-laden nature of continued injecting – may be necessary, as may changes in the approach to prescribing. Drug users will need regular medical input to monitor health and to deal with any illnesses as early as possible. They may also need help with other aspects of their lives – with their social lives, with housing or with welfare benefits – to try to maximise their chances of staying well (Green 1988b).

Typically, positive individuals need most help soon after being informed of the diagnosis. However, they also may need continuing help over a long period. The best way to provide a service may be through a mixture of regular appointments to monitor progress and encouraging the client to make contact whenever he or she has particular problems.

COUNSELLING THOSE WITH AIDS

Counselling those with AIDS is a complex process. Because no two people react in the same way to becoming ill with a disease which is likely to cause their death, it is not possible to think in terms of a 'typical case'. People react differently to AIDS as they react differently to other things in their lives (Miller 1987).

For virtually everyone with AIDS the diagnosis comes as a shock. Because of the nature of the disease people with AIDS often feel that they have lost control of their lives and the feeling increases if physical ill health begins to curtail their lives. However, loss of control is not inevitable. One of the key elements in counselling those with AIDS is helping them to start to sort out some of their problems, both problems they had before AIDS and also the new problems which having the disease brings them.

People with AIDS often require a good deal of practical as well as psychological support (George 1988). However good the counselling may be, it will not lead to well-being if the person with AIDS has nowhere to live or not enough to eat.

The particular difficulty which runs through the whole area of the counselling of the drug user with AIDS, or even the asymptomatic, is that the client has a dual problem – the problem of AIDS/HIV and the problem of drug abuse. In addition, the range of social problems, poor housing, lack of income and lack of social support which affect the drug user do so to a far greater extent than any other population at risk from HIV. With the drug user with AIDS, it is not possible to deal with the problems associated with HIV in isolation: counselling needs to deal with the whole person with all their problems; to attempt to do otherwise is a recipe for disaster.

REFERENCES

George H. (1988) 'Counselling people with AIDS, their lovers, friends and relations', in J. Green and A. McCreaner (eds) *Counselling in HIV Infection and AIDS*, London: Blackwell Scientific.

Green, J. (1986) 'Counselling HTLV-III Seropositives', in D. Miller, J. Weber and J. Green (eds) *Management of AIDS Patients*, London: Macmillan Press.

Green, J. (1988a) 'Post-test counselling', in J. Green and A. McCreaner (eds) *Counselling in HIV Infection and AIDS*, London: Blackwell Scientific.

Green, J. (1988b) 'Problem solving', in J. Green and A. McCreaner (eds) *Counselling in HIV Infection and AIDS*, London: Blackwell Scientific.

Green, J. (1989) 'Counselling in HIV infection and AIDS', in D. Miller, J. Weber and J. Green (eds) *Management of HIV Infection*, London: Macmillan Press.

Green, J. and McCreaner, A. (eds) (1988) *Counselling in HIV Infection and AIDS*, London: Blackwell Scientific.

McCreaner, A. (1988) 'Pre-test counselling', in J. Green and A. McCreaner (eds) *Counselling in HIV Infection and AIDS*, London: Blackwell Scientific.

McCreaner, A. (1989) 'Pre-test counselling', in D. Miller, J. Weber and J. Green (eds) *Management of HIV Infection*, London: Macmillan Press.

Miller, D. (1987) *Living with AIDS and HIV*, London: Macmillan Press.

Miller, R. and Bor, R. (1988) *AIDS: A Guide to Clinical Counselling*, London: Science Press.

Mulleady, G. (1988) 'Drug abuse and HIV', in J. Green and A. McCreaner (eds) *Counselling in HIV Infection and AIDS*, London: Blackwell Scientific.

Namir, S. (1986) 'Treatment issues concerning persons with AIDS', in L. McKusick (ed) *What to Do about AIDS*, Berkeley: University of California Press.

Schoenbaum, E.E., Davenney, K.S. and Selwyn, P.A. (1988) 'The impact of pregnancy on HIV-related disease', in C.N. Hudson and F. Sharp (eds) *AIDS and Obstetrics and Gynaecology*, London: Royal College of Obstetricians and Gynaecologists.

Chapter Twenty-two

MODELS OF SELF-HELP FOR DRUG USERS WITH HIV/AIDS

BILL NELLES

Many self-help organisations in the drug field focus on individuals acknowledging themselves to be dependent and vulnerable, in need of the critical perceptions and support of others. One of the strengths of self-help is its track record in encouraging and helping to sustain positive behaviour change amongst current and former drug-using individuals.

Nowadays, this goal is not only a crucial part of drug rehabilitation work, but of support for those who are HIV positive. Many drug users need to make radical changes in their behaviour, either to avoid infection by HIV or, if infected, to stay healthy and avoid infecting others. Self-help groups for drug users living with HIV and AIDS are forming all over the world, following the example set by the gay community.

The advent of the HIV epidemic has profoundly disturbed traditional forms of interaction between rehabilitation workers and clients. These same forces are also changing traditional patterns of self-help for drug users. There is now a greater appreciation of the need to respond to the spectrum of different problems that affect our clients, who are far from a homogeneous group. Chaotic injectors, stable methadone addicts, former (or 'recovering') drug users, and those on antagonist therapies – the needs of any two such individuals are often very different. The needs of one 'group' can no longer take priority over the needs of the other.

Existing models of self-help for people with AIDS taken from the gay community have shown themselves to be unrealistic for many drug users with AIDS (Nelles 1988). The health education literature and awareness-raising initiatives of these groups contributed much in the early days. However, fluent in taking a stand against the portrayal of homosexuality as an 'illness' or a deviation, some groups sought to import liberationist philosophy and politics from an arena where it was arguably appropriate, to addiction, where it was generally inappropriate and sometimes destructive.

Some gay men have perceived drug users as either a stereotyped group of criminals and psychological misfits, to be politely shunted off to special facilities or, more fraternally, as another persecuted minority. Both points of view are distortions. Many gay self-help groups have always operated programmes based on a notion of equality, rejecting traditional client/counsellor roles and allowing the individual to alternate between being a person in need of help, and a person giving help. When applied in the drug field, this has sometimes worked well – especially with recovering/ex-drug users – but at other times clients and workers have become confused by the shifting roles. In addition, this way of working assumes all members can consistently participate. Many current drug users sadly lack the stability in life to contribute in this particular way. Some members of gay-founded/orientated groups have found it hard to understand how messed up someone taking drugs can get. Telling someone who feels compelled to inject themselves with powerful substances that it is their right to do so and that their life-style is as valid as any other (as has been known to happen) does not help clients to overcome what any objective observer would see as a problem. The effect is rather to reinforce the most negative aspects of a drug-dependent life-style. Groups where this attitude predominated nearly veered away from a support and therapy role to that of a 'users' rights' stance, where the client's definition of what he or she needed was accepted without challenge. Challenge invited accusations of being prejudiced and patronising, not only from the clients but sometimes also from one's colleagues. In some circumstances this meant that the vulnerability of someone still dependent on drugs and their potential to get into deep water went unnoticed. People still dependent on drugs and struggling to cope with a diagnosis of HIV infection should neither be rejected as 'not one of us', nor saddled with the added burden of being confused by dubious rhetoric about freedom of life-styles.

Naturally, some drug users wanted to work as they saw the gay men working, whilst also attending for counselling; and some clients did this very successfully. However, many were not yet and perhaps never would be at the point where they could stop seeking and start giving help. This realisation is often painful for drug users, and needs to be handled sensitively if further alienation and damage to the self-esteem of all involved is to be avoided.

Whatever their mistakes, these early AIDS groups held the bridge for a long time while drug treatment agencies were learning the realities of AIDS. For that, many clients were and still are grateful. AIDS groups are now learning about drugs work, but still need to find out how to bring it into the mainstream of their activities.

MODELS OF SELF-HELP

There are, broadly speaking, three 'models' of HIV support groups that have evolved over the last two years in response to the epidemic in drug users. They might be loosely categorised as the 'junkies' union' approach, the 'separatist' approach and the 'coalition' approach.

The 'junkies' union' approach

These groups comprise drug users who are still actively involved in drug-taking and who act as a pressure group in support of their own rights. They are largely confined to the Netherlands (the *junkiebonden*) and some local areas in the UK. As the title suggests, these are associations for those who identify themselves as active drug users. The organisation acts as a focus for dialogue between those users still committed to their habit, and health care providers.

For many professionals, this type of organisation is unpalatable, as they see it as a forum 'promoting' drug use. This concern is to some extent justified. Clinically, it is highly undesirable for those who are HIV infected to continue injecting drugs, whether licit or illicit. This taboo is lacking in a 'junkies' union' model, whose participants may see little wrong with their life-style.

Supporters of this approach counter by insisting that the junkie's union operates more like a 'self-policing' force in the subculture, encouraging responsible behaviour in changing syringe and needle sharing behaviour. Indeed, it was the junkies' union' in the Netherlands that pioneered the successful Dutch needle-exchange system, which is now being copied in many cities. The Netherlands also has an enviable record in contacting 'street' users, and encouraging them into entering some form of treatment – as many as 70 per cent of the Amsterdam drug users are seen frequently, giving professionals opportunities to intervene (see Chapter 14). In the absence of the 'junkies' union' and its influence, it is unlikely that these programmes would have been so successful in attaining their goals.

Thus, the major problem with such organisations rests in their tendency to develop into 'users' rights' groups. Those who are drug-free, or disenchanted with drug use then find little in the group to their advantage and possibly some to their disadvantage (see Stamford 1989).

The 'separatist' approach

In these groups, ongoing drug users and ex-users do not work in the same group. Professional facilitators are sometimes involved. These groups have usually emerged from already established networks, such as Narcotics Anonymous, or from therapeutic communities. They are often abstinence-orientated. Gender has also played a part; in some areas, 'women only' groups have been established.

Often philosophies for coping with HIV infection are developed from the 'root' philosophy that underpins the group's views on drug use and abstinence. Concepts are already familiar to clients from their drug treatment, and the risk of the client feeling pulled between conflicting philosophies is minimised.

The main challenge for such groups is to avoid becoming too rigid in the expectations placed on clients. In some groups, the issue of members being prescribed narcotic analgesia or hypnotic medication has led to divisiveness. In some instances, clients who relapse can find themselves cut off from others in the group, triggering damaging feelings of rejection for the person concerned. However, other participants understandably fear that the safety of the group as a drug-free forum could be compromised.

The 'coalition' approach

In an attempt to counter the problem of operating from a

perspective that condones drug use, and being aware of the necessity of addressing the needs of several subgroups in the subculture, other groups have sought to combine support for drug users with a tolerant but limiting line on drug use itself. In these groups, the individual is expected to be somewhere in the continuum of treatment (but should not be injecting illicit street drugs). Whilst some operate separate groups for drug-free and drug-using clients, others run meetings in which the participants are either drug-free or 'stable' methadone users.

Access to professional facilitation is crucial, and must be accepted by all participants. Mixing of those who are drug-free and those whose drug use is reasonably stable may then be productive. The influence of non-users can be significant on those still on medication – provided the non-users understand that in the face of AIDS, not everyone can sustain abstinence. It is accepted in these groups (but by no means advocated) that some participants may return to methadone use and that help at this time may be particularly important. Flexibility is important, as the aim is to support drug users, not to alienate them.

Establishing clear rules and limits is essential. In the Terrence Higgins Trust Drug Support Group, the following criteria were established:

> Those attending the group should have been reliably diagnosed as HIV infected.
> Everyone attending should be either drug-free or stabilised on medication, but not using street drugs or injecting. (This accepts, however, that people might relapse, and allows for some flexibility for a temporary 'slip'.)
> Anyone arriving obviously 'stoned' may be asked to leave at the group's discretion.
> Confidentiality is paramount, and emphasised.
>
> (Nelles *et al.* 1988)

A particularly sensitive question is whether groups should mix together patients in advanced stages of HIV disease with those who are HIV infected but well. To an extent, they mix already, especially in cities where the epidemic started early in the 1980s. But with ever grimmer statistics on the mortality rate of those infected, healthy participants may over-identify with those in advanced stages, feeling death to be inevitable. This can provide a rationale for some to resume drug use, undoing the benefit of their period of abstinence or control. Others, seeing people *in extremis*, rise to the challenge of staying healthy and support those not as fortunate as themselves. This is one particular area in which more detailed research is badly needed.

Some drug-free clients may feel that they still want a forum that is abstinent, using the mixed group as a way of giving support and positive encouragement. In some organisations, former drug users aim to help not only 'stable' users but also more chaotic street users through a variety of 'outreach' schemes. Not only does the organisation offer counselling and group support, but health education and risk-reduction initiatives. They have avoided becoming 'right to use' pressure groups by the nature of their method of operation, that of professional and client working together.

Groups who have pioneered this model include ADAPT in New York City and the Terrence Higgins Trust Drug Support Group in the UK (Nelles *et al.* 1988). More recently, the UK organisation Mainliners has been created by a joint initiative involving 'professionals' and 'clients' working together in a spirit of co-operation and mutual respect (Palliser 1988). Initiatives such as this attract funding as they have the support of professionals who can lobby on their behalf.

The complex subject of how best to support and sustain those drug users who become infected with HIV is largely uncharted terrain. Self-help and its ability to sustain people making difficult changes in behaviour make it a vital area of development in the future.

REFERENCES

Nelles, W. (1988) 'Groups for HIV positive drug users', *DrugLink* 3(5): 9–10.

Nelles, W., Hogarth, S., Riccio, M. and Mulleady, G. (1988) 'The THT Drug Users Support Group', *DrugLink* 3(5): 11.

Palliser, I. (1988) 'Mainliners', *DrugLink*, 3(5): 10.

Stamford, C. (1989) 'Amsterdam revisited', *Mainliners* 2: 5.

Chapter Twenty-three

HIV POSITIVITY AND HEALTH IN THE THERAPEUTIC COMMUNITY

LESLEY COOKE, ANNETTE BARRATT AND DAVID TOMLINSON

THE ORIGINS OF THE THERAPEUTIC COMMUNITY

There is a relatively longstanding tradition in the United Kingdom of communities coming together to solve common problems. This has usually meant the more affluent and established members of that community providing goods and services for its disadvantaged poor. The almshouse and charitable hospitals were directly descended from this tradition. The moral outrage that the Victorians began to feel about poverty, death and disease amongst their underclass led to the founding of great institutions, amongst them the asylums. Whilst time or care in the community has overtaken this form of treatment, we only have to look at their imperious architecture to conclude that lofty ideals were involved in their creation.

Developments in medicine and the move to a more egalitarian society led ultimately to the greatest achievement of the post-war Labour government, the establishment of the National Health Service.

With these great traditions in our background and a health service that was to become the single largest employer in the country, it is interesting to note that in dealing with addictions in a non-medical context, we looked outside – most notably, to the United States – for the theoretical models of care. Any paper on residential rehabilitation that ignores the work of Maxwell Jones (1952) and his colleagues at the Maudsley Hospital, at the Henderson and at Dingleton on the Borders, does so at its peril; and it is widely acknowledged that Howard Bridger coined the expression 'therapeutic community'. Nevertheless, at a national and international level, the vast majority of services in the fields of alcohol and drug dependence owe their conception to a quite different tradition, one that is clearly anchored in the ideas of Bill W. and Dr Bob and their founding of Alcoholics Anonymous, which first met in 1935. The work of Alcoholics Anonymous and similar organisations – Narcotics Anonymous, Al-Anon and Fam-Anon – is well documented.

Two quite distinct forms of residential rehabilitation treatment grew out of Alcoholics Anonymous (AA). One is best known as the 'Minnesota Method' and adheres to the stepped programme (*The 12 Steps* 1987) and traditions of AA, while the other had its roots in the Synanon Foundation which based its practice on the family concept of AA. This was later imitated and adapted by Daytop Village and Phoenix House in New York City (De Leon and Ziegenfuss 1986).

It was from these two latter organisations that the world movement of therapeutic community care of drug takers evolved, and in an English setting the first organisation to put these ideas into practice was Alpha House, established in 1968 in Portsmouth. This was followed by Phoenix House in London, the Ley Community in Oxford, and Suffolk House in Slough on the edge of West London. While these agencies went on to develop in quite different ways, none the less there was (and still is) much common ground. This is now being seen with Minnesota Method Houses – the best known in the UK being Broadway Lodge and Clouds House, which became established during the 1980s.

DAWNING RECOGNITION OF HIV

With the advent of HIV, therapeutic communities suddenly found themselves in a situation which tested capabilities in many new and strenuous ways (Dickson and Hollis 1988). HIV, ARC and AIDS present the greatest challenge to the therapeutic movement since its inception. The challenge has many facets – moral, personal, medical and in terms of practice. Not all therapeutic communities have approached the issues in a thorough or open manner. Some have demanded pre-entry HIV test results and have refused places to those applicants who have been HIV positive. This has no doubt arisen from the massive fear and prejudice which have surrounded the disease and the virus. However, with the rapid spread of HIV amongst our client group, if the therapeutic community movement wishes to continue, it must adapt or die. For this reason, Phoenix House considered how to develop existing policy and practice at its four centres in England. This led to the realisation that some of the inadequacies could be met only by the creation of a specifically designed and resourceful service.

THE THERAPEUTIC COMMUNITY: DESCRIPTION OF OPERATION

There is much common ground between rehabilitation centres. Phoenix House retains the typical graduated programme and structure of a therapeutic community (Ogborne and Melotte 1977), although over the years it has softened and changed the style of therapy. It has moved away from major confrontation and encounter and has put greater emphasis on individual decision-making with support, rather than group decision-making.

Induction

On admission residents join 'Induction' for two to three months and do not leave the house unless accompanied by a senior resident or staff member. During this period people are able to 'find their feet' by learning how the programme is working and by developing social relationships. These processes are encouraged by their peers, senior residents and staff; fellow residents within the induction group constitute the peer group and many friendships are formed which last beyond the programme. This is perhaps more important for those with HIV because of the possibility of greater physical and emotional dependence on others. The cementing of friendships throughout the programme establishes the support which is an invaluable source of comfort and reassurance in times of crisis, particularly once people are living independently.

Phase 1

The first six months are very demanding. Apart from group work, one-to-one counselling, educational seminars and leisure activities, residents in Phase 1 are expected to run the house and are allocated to a department such as catering or gardens. Residents can work their way up the hierarchy within their department, gaining promotion as they would in an employment situation. They can also request a move to other departments. The staff role at this stage is to determine how the needs of the individual can best be met within the programme. Staff closely involve and consult the more senior residents who have an important supervisory role in the community.

Phase 2

After six to eight months, residents usually request to move to Phase 2. This is still based within the main house, but the resident is free to go out from the house unescorted and to have time in the evenings to do as he or she chooses. During the day residents participate in the programme on a standard nine-to-five basis, working alongside staff assisting with decision-making both on practical and clinical matters. Phase 2 is a time when people are expected to consider their future and they are encouraged to develop and strengthen their links with the outside world. Traditionally, this has meant pursuing vocational experience through voluntary work at least one day per week, and organising options for training or education, which in turn necessitates dealing with organisations and getting involved in social and personal relationships in 'straight' society.

Phase 3 and Re-entry

Phase 3 is the final stage in preparing to return to the wider world. This is one of the more testing times for people; it is when they move out of the main house and live in the smaller re-entry house with minimal staff supervision. Here the individual can make decisions around issues such as alcohol, and residents usually decide to follow a controlled drinking model or abstain. There is greater freedom to explore relationships and leisure interests. Residents are assisted by the staff in seeking employment or educational courses and a housing assessment is carried out to identify appropriate move-on accommodation. In Phase 3 or Re-entry, people share household tasks and negotiate together to establish their own boundaries and rules for communal living.

During this time residents are still expected to adhere to a drug-free philosophy and other programme expectations relating to independent living skills. They attend one or two group meetings a week so that staff can assess how they are coping and offer any support needed. Residents are encouraged to talk through their anxieties about the future, and through a combination of practical and emotional assistance they are usually ready to move on in approximately six months. There is still the opportunity to return weekly for a group meeting attended by those who have left the programme. This is initially for a period of six months but is extendable if necessary.

RE-EXAMINING OUR PRACTICE

Since 1984 the Phoenix Houses in the UK have admitted clients who are HIV positive. Over that time policies have evolved to accommodate the needs of these clients. Many issues arose in trying to adapt Phoenix House so as to accommodate the special needs of those with HIV.

Health and safety

An urgent check of existing health and safety policies was undertaken because it was obviously of paramount importance to create a safe environment in which the spread of the virus would be prevented. This would reassure staff and residents alike. The families of those working and living at Phoenix House were in many cases initially concerned about health risks posed by HIV-positive residents to their loved ones. This was in turn compounded by the fact that approximately half of the staff are ex-drug users and have their own fears arising from previous needle-sharing and drug-related relationships. The shock of HIV and AIDS on staff personally cannot be underestimated. It precipitated a state of denial in some staff which made it impossible for them to support residents. Health and safety policies covering the more contagious Hepatitis B were extended, particularly in relation to cleaning body fluid spillages, the disposal of soiled waste and the covering of broken skin.

The potential for sexual transmission of the virus raised a dilemma in the therapeutic community: sexual relationships are discouraged for various reasons but it was decided condoms should be made available regardless.

Through a series of factual seminars and training sessions we were able to allay staff and residents' fears relating to infection, and provide information on safer sex practices and other preventative measures. The sessions also provided opportunities to express personal concerns and attitudes regarding the virus and working with those who are HIV positive. Fortnightly staff groups on the subject have since been formalised and discussion points range from how to cope with clients using analgesics (the philosophy advocates abstinence from all drugs) through to whether the spot-check urine sampling should be continued.

Policy and practice on HIV testing and confidentiality

In the initial stages people were encouraged to have a test and blood could be taken on the premises by the visiting medical or paramedical staff along with pre- and post-test counselling. It was realised that this compromised individuals who felt pressurised to have a test, yet did not help staff or residents in coming to terms with the result. When testing was first available people were naive about its consequences. Many of the staff offered to be tested, in some cases primarily to be of moral support to the residents. They were advised against this course of action because of possible discrimination in areas such as employment and insurance. Those awaiting test results were in a compromised and public situation. Consequently, the system was changed to one of personal responsibility. It is now up to the individual whether to be tested and whether to reveal the result or not. Residents can attend any special clinic for this purpose. It was recognised that the sensible way forward for effective health and safety was to assume everyone at the project – residents and staff alike – to be HIV positive. All those entering are informed accordingly, as are all health professionals involved with Phoenix House.

Confidentiality is a major, problematic issue when rehabilitating people back into the community. Facilitating a good, consistent primary health care service from GPs, hospitals and dentists needs careful consideration and negotiation. Following bad experiences, it is now the Phoenix House practice to check how a statutory or voluntary agency keeps its documentation and who has access to it in order to advise residents regarding disclosure of confidential information. The health service is not the main offender in this respect; the lack of procedures in local government and the benefit system is frightening. When they are about to make the final step to independence, HIV-positive residents find that in order to gain suitable housing and enhanced income, it is sometimes necessary to reveal their status and even to provide medical confirmation. Those who have chosen not to have a test or who wish to keep information confidential are put at a disadvantage. Therefore, staff must make it part of their role to educate other agencies about confidentiality.

Confidentiality within the house is designed for the purposes of resident and staff support. If a resident discloses his or her HIV status to a member of staff it is treated as a team responsibility, and discussed as part of the clinical meeting. A 'team' represents the group of staff responsible for each different part of the programme. This is preferable to the information being confidential to the individual team member, because it not only provides a consistent, appropriate network for the resident, but it also prevents the stress falling on one member of staff who may feel isolated with such knowledge, unable to discuss it with colleagues for fear of breaking worker/client confidentiality. It also prevents a resident putting undue pressure on individual staff members, which could be onerous in these circumstances.

Staff support and conditions

It is preferable for the therapeutic community staff not to have the responsibility of pre- and post-test counselling. Staff are generally neither specifically trained in this type of counselling, nor trained in working with clients with a life-threatening disease. Much has been provided in the way of information, advice, training and support, primarily through external professionals. This does not change the fact that HIV and its related illnesses can be disturbing for the non-medically trained and those not confident in their sensitivity around the issues of bereavement.

HIV has major implications for personnel policy and planning, both at local management level (in the form of staff recruitment, training and support) and at an organisational level (in the form of equal opportunities, staff sickness and 'burn-out'). It has been possible to address these issues in new facilities, but existing projects not planned with HIV in mind are hidebound by insufficiently flexible funding.

With regard to equal opportunities, HIV has not caused Phoenix House to change its practice of employing ex-drug users to run the programme. If a job applicant or employee discloses their HIV-antibody-positive status, this information is held in strictest confidence but does not prejudice their situation. In anticipation of increased staff sickness it is essential to build a higher level of sickness leave into the budget. The problem of cross-infection to immune-suppressed clients will also necessitate this. The extra sick-time allowance reduces pressure felt by those having to cover for absent colleagues. This helps prevent overwork and 'burn-out' in combination with specialists within the staff complement whose role is to facilitate staff support groups and provide advice and counselling as requested by staff on an individual basis.

Changes in the programme

The programme content needed changing as a result of HIV to a less intense approach. Diet, relaxation, safer sex and personal care have been incorporated as important aspects of the therapeutic community so as to encourage people to develop a healthy life-style. This was effected across the board for all residents. At a later stage of adapting the programme, clients who had disclosed a positive test result began to request additional support groups specifically to discuss the feelings created by this. These were facilitated by staff after extra training from recently established self-help groups outside the therapeutic community (see Chapter 22).

The process has not always been smooth. For example, other residents sometimes feel that the HIV-positive group are being given priority, and there have been cases where residents wishing to avoid certain responsibilities have feigned illness.

Staff have also felt vulnerable when a resident has suddenly become ill. Whereas previously they used their own common sense in caring for residents who were displaying symptomatology of minor complaints, they are now more concerned about misjudging the situation. This fear of misjudgement relates to other aspects of the programme, as when residents have not lived up to staff expectations.

If expectations become too low, through the fear of creating stress and exacerbating illness, the programme may become ineffective; a client may then feel that his or her drug problem is not being addressed and may choose to leave the programme. This places greater stress on staff because their decision-making is more vital. The problem was eased by a special staff support group with an outside facilitator specifically for the purpose of talking through these issues. It allowed staff the opportunity not only to discuss residents' programme assessment and planning in the light of HIV, but also their own feelings on sexuality, death and illness.

The first residents with ARC caused some considerable perturbation by the speed with which they became profoundly ill. The staff are not medically trained (although some do have a practical nursing background) and found it difficult to manage if more than one or two at a time became ill. The therapeutic community is not designed for the needs of those becoming unwell, there is no mobility access and all bedrooms are on the first floor with no lift. Within the current structure, as more people need active physical care, the self-help principle based on full and active participation quickly becomes unworkable. A facility is required which is physically designed and appropriately resourced for those who are too unwell to use the existing programme but want more than ever before to tackle their addiction.

THE NEW APPROACH FOR THE NEW HOUSE

An example of such a response is the new special house being set up by Phoenix House in London. Intended for those who are HIV positive and unwell, it comprises 25 residents in the main house and ten in the annexe. The annexe will accommodate those who are preparing to move back into the community and those who, as a result of ARC or AIDS, have been rendered homeless or are at risk of relapse into drug addiction. When we began developing this project, we soon realised that it was unique and many questions had to be answered for which there were no tried and tested formulae.

Entry criteria

The first area warranting particular attention is the admissions procedure. Referrals will come from a broader spectrum of agencies; currently, drug users reach Phoenix House via street agencies, the courts, or other statutory and voluntary bodies. The individual has to make a direct contact with the admissions team, by whom they are then interviewed and the suitability of the programme assessed. The broader spectrum of referral agencies will include hospitals, out-patient clinics, housing associations and obviously other organisations working specifically with those with HIV disease.

Referrals from general practitioners are rare at present. However, if general practitioners respond positively to calls that they should take a more active role in relation to drug users and HIV, then we can expect an increase in referrals from this source (Advisory Council on the Misuse of Drugs 1989).

In determining suitability for the new project it was felt that some form of health evaluation would also be required as part of the initial assessment. The format of such an evaluation has not been finalised, but the extension has resource implications for the development of an appropriate service and we intend to identify general practitioner back-up sufficient to attend to the health needs of the residents. This could also include the possibility of assessments in prisons (see Chapter 18). At present, our admissions team interview applicants on remand and pre-parole, but lack training to determine their medical suitability for the programme. This begs the question as to the criteria for suitability in terms of health/ill health. HIV disease is not always predictable – not only may people become unwell very suddenly, but the reverse may also occur.

Dementia (see Chapter 5) is a whole new problem for therapeutic communities but one which is extremely pertinent in relation to the planned project. Once again we are trying to design a balanced model in terms of rehabilitative goals and the staffing necessary to achieve them. There may prove to be a stage at which the presentation of dementia would render the model unworkable. Therefore, these clients will be admitted with regard to the staff complement and the needs of the other residents.

The programme

In the new project the programme will need to be designed so as to provide a relevant service for those who are incapacitated. Although the basic concept of resident involvement in the running of the house will be maintained, extra staff – including cooks and domestic assistants – will be employed to ensure the work of the departments is lighter.

Knowledge of health as well as rehabilitation issues concerning drug use and HIV is intended to maximise creative thinking around appropriate life-styles. It is hoped this will encourage residents to reject drug use and its consequent damage to the body, replacing it with an increased awareness of how illness can be combated by taking good care of one's own physical, mental and emotional health. There will be an emphasis on diet, bearing in mind that drug users normally present with evidence of malnutrition. Good nourishment to combat infection is vital. In the later stages of HIV illness problems may arise such as difficulty in swallowing or soreness in the mouth (see Chapter 4). Diarrhoea or nausea and vomiting due to HIV illness or as a side-effect of treatment also draw attention to the need for expert advice on nutrition. For these reasons we envisage appointing a professional dietician. The staff will have more time to develop information and expertise in alternative therapies and a health educationalist will be appointed to promote health, stress reduction, safer sex and a general positive outlook; we hope to be able to make available a range of options for 'healing', both within the house and via outside amenities.

For many of those with HIV, ARC or AIDS, Phase 2 of the programme has been a time to develop the self-help concept. They have become a resource for the field in general by providing training, information and structured volunteer support. This is also a time when people explore what can be offered by social services, other voluntary organisations and possibly the community nursing service.

The new project will also develop Phoenix House's role in facilitating any reconciliation residents may wish between themselves and friends and relatives. Many such relationships have been destroyed through drug use. The implications of working with the family and/or partners will be far greater, because of the complexity of emotions derived from having a loved one with such a stigmatising and life-threatening illness. Therefore, expertise in this area has been incorporated into the staff complement, including bereavement counselling experience and training.

Moving out of the house

The move away from the main house into the annexe of the new project is partly designed to give residents a realistic idea of the services available to people with HIV, ARC or AIDS in the community. Community nurses will take responsibility for day-to-day nursing care, as they would do if the residents were in their own home. This is an excellent opportunity for the resident to experience for the first time the actual workings of such an arrangement. It provides the opportunity to discuss and resolve any difficulties this might cause, rather than feeling isolated, panic-stricken and unable to cope with the situation at a later stage. It is also our intention to ensure, if a resident would like a 'buddy' or helper (see Chapter 22), that they can try out different personnel or arrangements, so that unnecessary trauma is prevented at a later time. If people express a wish to be sited near each other or to share accommodation once they leave, every effort will be made to achieve this. Leavers are encouraged to return for social and community events.

The enhancement of good health and the accessibility of services will be a major focus of the resettlement workers. Their role will also facilitate support from statutory and voluntary bodies as desired by the individual, as well as co-ordinate support from Phoenix House.

Over the past three years it has become progressively more difficult to find housing for our residents. The annexe has been designed with a dual purpose in mind, not only to provide accommodation for the re-entrants but also to offer the flexibility to take in past clients who are at risk of relapse for various reasons, such as coming to terms with ARC or AIDS, homelessness, fear of harassment or poor health. Thus, there is much concern about the inadequate availability of suitable accommodation for people with HIV disease. Phoenix House has recently become registered as a housing association in its own right, which will enable it to plan better for the future in this area of under-provision.

CONCLUSION

Over the years the expertise of therapeutic communities in rehabilitating people to a drug-free life has become well recognised by government and its representative bodies both in the UK and worldwide. In order to develop appropriate responses to HIV within the therapeutic community, it has to be recognised that this is a difficult and painful process, and can only be successful where the determination exists. The therapeutic community movement is responding to the challenge of HIV and the choice of freedom from addiction for those infected is a choice it aims to preserve.

REFERENCES

Advisory Council on the Misuse of Drugs (1989) *AIDS and Drug Misuse Report: Part II*, London: HMSO.

De Leon, G. and Ziegenfuss, J.T. (eds) (1986) *Therapeutic Communities for Addictions: Readings in Theory, Research and Practice*, Springfield, Illinois: Charles C. Thomas.

Dickson, S. and Hollis, J. (1988) 'AIDS in the house', *DrugLink* 3(2): 12–13.

Jones, M. (1952) *Social Psychiatry: The Therapeutic Community*, London: Tavistock Publications.

Ogborne, A.C. and Melotte, C. (1977) 'An evaluation of a therapeutic community for former drug users', *British Journal of Addiction* 72: 75–82.

The 12 Steps (1987), San Diego, California: Recovery Publications.

Chapter Twenty-four

PRIMARY CARE: THE CHALLENGE OF HIV INFECTION TO THE CARE OF THE DRUG TAKER

RICHARD ELION

The primary care of the drug taker is a challenging task that requires great resources, and even greater flexibility. Hospital-based specialist services are not able to provide treatment for all HIV-positive drug takers – nor would it be entirely acceptable to the patient population even if they were able to do so. It is essential that primary health care services are developed so that they can provide a wider range of services, at time of need and in a local setting, to this group who have for so long failed to utilise health services adequately and to receive essential health care.

Primary care should be the drug taker's major route to health care, and can be their first and most consistent point of contact with the health system. It should address their psychological needs related to addiction and also their medical needs. Primary care provides a framework of health for the client. The critical aspect in its delivery is the understanding that the patient's needs are often only indirectly related to their health status. The delivery of care must be user-sensitive, culturally specific and readily available. The client should feel respected and cared for and be able to discuss their addiction and medical problems without fears of judgement.

The need to work with injecting drug users in a primary care setting has never been greater. They are at high risk for exposure to HIV as a result of their sharing of needles and syringes. In addition, they are likely to have sexual contacts with other drug users, thereby further increasing their risk. This population also is the most important reservoir of viral exposure for perinatal spread, and a key portal of entry into the non-drug-using heterosexual population through contact with prostitutes and other sexual partners. The challenge of working with substance abusers must stimulate effective health strategies for empowering them to improve their health care and reduce their risk of acquiring and spreading HIV.

The medical issues in the care of the substance abusing population are intimately connected to that population's addictive behaviour. The care of these individuals has been delegated to the substance-abuse field, which is expected to assume all care for this population. This is not a practical solution. The ability to care for the medical needs of substance abusers greatly exceeds the capacity of the substance-abuse field. It creates a prejudicial form of health care for primary care to shun the needs of such a large population.

Primary care must be comprehensive, if it is to be effective. The illnesses of addiction and HIV infection must be treated simultaneously. An effective approach demands recognition of how these illnesses are related, so that clients' health needs are congruent with their care. The clinician should co-ordinate the medical and addictive aspects of care. AIDS is a primary care function, not the province of subspecialists.

The first section of this chapter will describe the psychosocial aspects of primary care for substance abusers and present critical areas of focus for the practitioner in working with this population. The second section will focus on medical care issues and the conclusion will make recommendations for health policy relating to primary care and substance abuse.

THE PSYCHOSOCIAL ASPECTS OF PRIMARY CARE

The first maxim of primary care for drug takers is *flexibility and a supportive, non-judgemental approach.* Working with drug takers causes anxiety among health providers. Injecting drug takers are often blamed for their plight and may not receive compassionate care. Some facilities present various procedural obstacles to the clients, such as observing waiting times or appointment times which are normal for most patients but impossible for addicted individuals. The health facilities must be flexible and resourceful enough to adapt to the different needs of the individuals and not necessarily demand that they fit into all of the institutional limitations.

The second maxim of primary health care for this population is the *prevention of new exposures to the virus and decreasing the risk of subsequent transmission and spread.* This is the prime public health objective and focuses efforts on education and counselling of the injecting drug user. Many researchers have documented the educability of this community (see Chapter 16) and question the long-term changes of these self-protective behaviours (see review by Becker and Joseph 1988; and Chapter 8).

Sixty per cent of drug takers seem receptive to interventions aimed at bringing about changes in their behaviour. The figure of 60 per cent is fairly consistent through different studies of behaviour change in this population. The remaining 40 per cent are quite resistant to change and difficult to reach. This is further complicated by the findings that the majority of first-time users share needles on their first experience (Des Jarlais and Friedman 1988). Future work to change injecting practice must reach the client before the first injection, so these efforts must obviously also occur outside of treatment programmes. The primary care contact may provide such an early opportunity for education.

There is no medical reason for compulsory testing. The third maxim is that *in the care of the individual, testing for HIV status should be used with a specific clinical goal, such as establishing a diagnosis, or entering a research trial with informed consent.* This process takes a great deal of time and must be incorporated into a comprehensive programme to ensure therapeutic benefit for the client. HIV antibody testing is currently available to the primary health practitioner. It is the meeting point between education and medical care. In one study of clients in a methadone maintenance programme, 72 per cent were in favour of a voluntary HIV screening programme but only 50 per cent were in favour of these results being available to the clinical staff.

There are certain clinical situations where the antibody result might help to establish a diagnosis for a patient. A patient with TB would be classified with AIDS, according to the Centers for Disease Control criteria, if the individual was antibody positive (see Chapter 4). The test result might point out the need for an immunological work-up in certain situations or direct the investigation in a particular direction, depending on the individual patient. A seropositive test may affect decisions concerning antiviral therapy for some patients as well.

There may be potential conflicts between the patient's need for confidentiality and privacy and the clinical benefits that might result from identifying serological status. Patients may be afraid to know their status, and may become suicidal on learning of a positive result. They may not want the result on their medical records for fear of discrimination. The test results may cause greater risk behaviour in certain individuals, as they attempt to self-medicate in response to a significant stressor.

The fourth maxim concerns *the need for long-term supportive counselling*. The psychosocial aspects of HIV testing are clearly important to the subsequent attitude of the individual. This is important, regardless of the test outcome. It must be reinforced that someone who is seronegative could convert in time and the need for precautions remains in effect despite the negative result. The seropositive individual will obviously need continuous support as well. The use of group dynamics in combination with individual counselling is beneficial.

The psychosocial demands of this group change as HIV illness progresses. Many individuals develop different stages of dementia and may have specific neurological complaints as well (see Chapter 5). Approximately 30 to 40 per cent also develop cognitive difficulties, making it more difficult to provide counselling and medical support. The extra questions and confusion by the drug taker may reflect cognitive or neurological difficulties rather than an intoxicated drug state. Care and specificity must be given to specific diagnoses as they relate to psychological affect, to distinguish these changes from HIV-related causes, anxiety or drug dependence.

THE MEDICAL ASPECTS OF PRIMARY CARE

The primary medical care of drug takers should be integrated into the addiction treatment whenever possible. Close linkages with health clinics outside the drug programmes are acceptable but must provide easy access and flow of information between programmes. The care of an HIV-positive patient is best handled by a primary care provider and only requires specialists in few specific circumstances. The provider should understand the symptoms associated with AIDS such as fever, lymphadenopathy, shortness of breath, diarrhoea and headache and know how to initiate appropriate diagnostic studies (see Chapters 3 and 4).

Infections such as cellulitis, endocarditis and pneumonia are often more prevalent in injecting drug takers and must be investigated effectively as well. Four areas will be highlighted below as they are common areas of HIV-related symptomatology.

The lungs

A major area of importance is infections of the lungs. There is an increased incidence of bacterial pneumonia in HIV-infected injectors. Also, there is a concomitant increase in mortality due to pneumonia among young adults. This is presumably due to the B-cell dysfunction that occurs in HIV infection and the subsequent weakness against encapsulated organisms.

The most common presentations of AIDS are pulmonary complaints. Sixty per cent of all HIV-positive patients will present with PCP (pneumocystis carinii pneumonia) as their initial opportunistic infection and more than 80 per cent of all AIDS patients will acquire PCP during their illness (Murray *et al.* 1987). The treatment of PCP is important for the primary care clinician and is not different from the standard treatments. These include cotrimoxazole (Bactrim, Septrin), pentamidine or trimetrexate or dapsone plus trimethoprim. The patient will require subsequent prophylaxis for PCP which could include intermittent dapsone, cotrimoxazole or aerosolised pentamidine. This treatment is also identical to the remainder of the HIV-infected populations.

There are significant other pulmonary infections such as simple bacterial pneumonia or mycobacterial infections. This may include mycobacterium tuberculosis (TB) or mycobacterium kansasii or mycobacterium avium (MAI). The diagnosis of these infections may be difficult as the usual test of exposure for TB, the intermediate-strength purified protein derivative (PPD) lacks sensitivity in seropositive patients and is seldom positive in end-stage HIV disease. A positive PPD may occur in patients with early HIV disease, but a negative result does not exclude the diagnosis of past exposure or even current disease. The clinician must therefore depend on the identification of acid-fast organisms. Anti-tubercular treatment should be withheld if possible until this has been documented (see Glatt *et al.* 1988).

The exact diagnosis of tuberculosis is often problematic. Analysis of the sputum of HIV-positive patients is less helpful than for non-HIV-infected patients in identification of the organism. It is frequently necessary to resort to brochoscopy or biopsy of lymph nodes, liver or bone marrow to establish the diagnosis. Occasionally, even those steps may not help as classical pathological changes of granuloma format might be minimal or absent. It is thought that this lack of test response may result from compromise of the immune system which is necessary in the formation of granulomas.

The majority of TB cases in AIDS patients occur in injecting drug takers from poor socio-economic areas and poor hygiene where TB is more prevalent. TB and other bacterial pneumonias seem to occur more frequently in injecting drug takers than other HIV-infected populations. These pneumonias may cause nearly equivalent morbidity as the more commonly recognised PCP infection.

The TB infection reflects the defects in cell-mediated immunity lowering the resistance to reactivation. This infection often precedes the classical diagnosis of AIDS. The presentation of TB is seldom simple in the drug taker, with limited extrapulmonary TB or disseminated disease being found in approximately 75 per cent of cases. The X-ray findings are often atypical with classical upper lobe disease and cavitation being the exception. The findings may be indistinguishable from other opportunistic infections which makes a pathological diagnosis essential. The treatment of TB is normally accomplished with the usual two-drug regimen of isoniazid and rifampin. These are often supplemented with streptomycin, ethambutol or pyrazinamide, or combinations depending on the sensitivities identified at culture. The exact duration of treatment is controversial, with regimens lasting from nine months to longer. Therapy should continue for at least six months after cultures become negative, but the exact duration for adequate therapy is not known. The treatment of MAI is much more problematic because there is no adequate cure and prolonged treatment may result in serious side-effects.

The bowel

The second area of particular interest in the care of injecting drug takers is the treatment of infections of the bowel. These include giardia lamblia, cryptosporidium and isospora belli. The latter two are protozoan infections which are very important in the care of this population. The treatments for these infections are not different than in other non-HIV-infected patients.

The Central Nervous System

The third area is the Central Nervous System which may be infected with bacterial meningitis or disseminated meningitis from cryptococcus neoformans, or toxoplasma gondii. The latter two are protozoan infections and are treated according to standard protocols (Goldschmidt *et al.* 1988). Other possible infections include syphilis, and there is the fear of missing untreated tertiary syphilis (Johns *et al.* 1987). The current recommendations from the CDC specify treatment of HIV-positive patients with a positive titre for the VDRL test for syphilis with the regimen for tertiary syphilis. The patient is retested with the VDRL titre after a suitable time, from three to six months. If the titre is still positive, a spinal tap should be performed and high-dose intravenous penicillin considered if the VDRL of the spinal fluid is positive.

Fungal infections

The fourth area relates more to a class of infections than a discrete physiological system. Fungal infections may be simple but they can be disturbing and may even be life-threatening. These range from oral candidiasis to meningitis secondary to cryptococcal infections. Clotrimazole troches or Nystatin suspension are usually adequate for oral infections. Ketroconazole 400 mg is often needed for refractory treatments and is usually sufficient for oesophageal candidiasis as well. Amphotericin B is reserved for cryptococcus infections and refractory oesophageal candidiasis as well, but only rarely needed for the latter.

THE USE OF ANTIVIRAL DRUGS IN THE PRIMARY CARE SETTING

Antiviral medications may be used as remittive therapy for HIV disease and as prophylactic therapy in combination with the PCP regimens mentioned earlier. Fischl *et al.* (1987) have demonstrated the significant decrease in the number and severity of opportunistic infections that results from administration of antiretroviral therapy. It is currently felt that additional prophylaxis for PCP is needed in addition to antiretroviral therapy to ensure adequate protection. The use of TMP/SMX and aerosolised pentamidine has been beneficial as prophylaxis. These medicines have been used with drug-misusing populations but have significant risks of haematological toxicity. It is important to ensure adequate follow-up by monitoring blood parameters to limit the side-effects as well as to monitor compliance. The patient who is taking adequate amounts of zidovudine (AZT) will display elevated MCV secondary to the drug. This would not appear to be a toxic side-effect and may be used as an additional monitor of compliance.

The care of this population is not simply putting people on the right medicines and following them properly. Practitioners need to understand the patient's goals and belief systems and meld the 'cures' in with the patient's own systems. Drug takers will frequently not take medicines that may interfere with their ability to use illicit substances (i.e. prevent their high). This is seen with medicines that increase the ability of the liver to metabolise other drugs, specifically for rifampin and phenobarbitone and some of the other anti-TB medicines as well. The patients feel the medication may prevent their high and therefore take it on an intermittent basis. This issue needs to be discussed in a risk/benefit context so as to enlist the patient's co-operation, rather than attempting to confront their logic.

PERINATAL CARE AND HIV INFECTION

Many injecting drug takers are women, virtually all of whom are of reproductive age. The care of these women and their pregnancies has become an important aspect of primary care with this population. It is critical to educate women who are possibly HIV positive about the risks of pregnancy – not only for themselves but also because of the 30–50 per cent risk of transmission of HIV to the newborn (Minkoff 1987). All practitioners should be comfortable discussing the option of termination of pregnancy with HIV-seropositive women and be able to describe the full implications of pregnancy for the women as well. In considering the factors relating to continuation or termination of pregnancy, the patient's decisions may relate more to social factors than medical factors and this perspective should be integrated into the counselling plan.

CONCLUSION

The growing need for care among HIV-infected people is overcrowding an overcrowded system. The needs of women addicts, their perinatal concerns and the concerns of their children create yet more stress on the system. The care of prisoners, the care of heterosexual contacts and their subsequent sexual contacts are all related to the needs of drug takers with HIV infection. It is not only uncaring but also lacking in foresight to ignore the needs of such a large segment of our population.

The solution is to create a model of primary care that is responsive to the issues of addiction. We must incorporate our own models of wellness with the patient's concept of wellness. This might include intermittent drug use or sporadic compliance with medication regimes, even though this does not fit in with the pattern that the clinician had designed. The goal, therefore, should be to maximise the health of the individual and create a model to which the drug taker can relate. The health institutions can and must create a network of care that is supportive for drug takers. The failure of the present network to engage this population is a damning indictment of our public health system – and it highlights the potentially serious repercussions for the population as a whole. It is a time for compassion and creativity as well as pragmatism: we must enlarge our network and respond to this pressing challenge.

REFERENCES

Becker, M.H. and Joseph, J.G. (1988) 'AIDS and behavioural change to reduce risk: a review', *American Journal of Public Health* 78: 394–410.

Des Jarlais, D.C. and Friedman, S.R. (1988) 'Needle sharing among IVDUs at risk for AIDS', *American Journal of Public Health* 78: 1496–9.

Fischl, M.A. *et al.* (1987) 'The efficacy of AZT in the treatment of patients with AIDS and AIDS-related complex: a double blind placebo controlled trial', *New England Journal of Medicine* 317: 185–91.

Glatt, A.E., Chirgwin, K., Lamdesman, S.H. (1988) 'Treatment of infections associated with Human Immunodeficiency Virus', *New England Journal of Medicine* 318(22): 1439–48.
Goldschmidt, R.H. *et al.* (1988) 'Evaluation and treatment of AIDS-associated illnesses: an approach for the primary physician', *Journal of the American Board of Family Practice* 1(2): 112–30.
Johns, D.R. *et al.* (1987) 'Alterations in the natural history of neurosyphilis by concurrent infection with the human immunodeficiency virus', *New England Journal of Medicine* 316: 1569–72.
Minkoff, H.L. (1987) 'Care of pregnant women infected with Human Immunodeficiency Virus', *Journal of the American Medical Association* 258: 2714–17.
Murray, J.E. *et al.* (1987) 'Pulmonary complications of the Acquired Immunodeficiency Syndrome: an update', *American Review of Respiratory Disease* 135: 504–9.

INDEX